Home Health Aide: Guidelines for Care

A Handbook for Caregiving at Home

Home Health Aide: Guidelines for Care

A Handbook for Caregiving at Home

SECOND EDITION

TINA M. MARRELLI
MSN, MA, RN

with assistance from:

SANDRA WHITTIER
RN, BC, MSN
Case Coordinator
VNA Care Network
Gloucester, Massachusetts

Printed in the United States of America.
Printing/binding by Fineline Graphics, Inc.

P.O. Box 629
Boca Grande, FL 33921
www.marrelli.com
news@marrelli.com

International Standard Book Number
13: 978-0-9647801-3-2

International Standard Book Number
10: 0-9647801-3-5

PREFACE & ACKNOWLEDGEMENT

This second edition (like the first), was inspired by home health and hospice aides and team members who are continually striving to help care for patients at home.

Like all books, input and motivation comes from many sources and often, over many years. First, thank you to all who have inspired me over many years –so many people in home health and hospice –thank you!

Special thanks to Laura Friend, BSN, RN Executive Director of the West Virginia Council of Home Health Agencies and Sandra Whittier, RN, BC, MSN for all of their input and assistance on the first editions of the aide books (handbook and instructor manual) and continued support and reviews of this second, revised edition.

Gratitude also to Lynda S. Hilliard, MBA, RN, Deloitte & Touche for her friendship, time, and instant feedback and at all hours! Finally, to Bill Glass and Limpy Buttercup Glass for their love and good humor. I could not do what I do without you!

REVIEWERS

Jane Cooperman, MS, RN, BC
Director of Clinical Services
Essex Valley Visiting Nurse Association
Newark, New Jersey

Jo Jo Dantone-DeBarbieris, MS, LDN, RD, CDE
President and CEO
Nutrition Education Resources, Inc.
LaPlace, Louisiana

Genie Eide, RN, BSN, CNA
Consultant
Home Health/Hospice Consulting Services, Inc.
Scottsdale, Arizona

Cindy Farris, MPH, BSN, RN
Medical Assistant Program Faculty Member
South College
Knoxville, Tennessee

Carroll Fernstrom,OTR/L
Occupational Therapist and Consultant
Raleigh, North Carolina

Anita Finkelman, MSN, RN
Consultant and Faculty
Cincinnati, Ohio

Laura Friend, BSN, RN
Executive Director
West Virginia Council of Home Health Agencies, Inc.
Middlebourne, West Virginia

Joie Glenn, RN, MBA
Executive Director
The New Mexico Association for Home Care
Albuquerque, New Mexico

Catherine Halsey, RN, CHPN
Hospital Care Coordinator
Tidewell Hospice and Palliative Care
Englewood, Florida

Margery Harvey-Griffith, MS, RN
Clinical Operations Consultant
Boca Raton, Florida

Karen Lamb, ND, RN, CS
Associate Professor of Nursing
Rush University Medical Center
Chicago, Illinois

Mary Marrelli, CNA
San Clemente, California

Sharon Newton, RN, PhD
Consultant
Healthcare ConsultLink
Fort Davis, Texas

Cathy Sasser, RPh
Operations Performance Manager
Critical Care Systems, Inc.
Atlanta, Georgia

Karen Suedkamp, RN, MSN, HCS-D
President
Suedkamp Enterprise, Inc.
Morrow, Ohio

Pamella Tynan
Regional Clinical Director
Odyssey Healthcare, Inc.
Dallas, Texas

Sandy Whittier, RN, BC, MSN
Case Coordinator
VNA Care Network
Gloucester, Massachusetts

Maureen Williams, MEd, RN, BC
Regional Director
Capital Hospice
Leesburg and Manassas, Virginia

CONTENTS

Appendix

GUIDELINES FOR USE

The goal of this book is to help home health and hospice aides and certified nursing assistants provide safe and effective care to their patients while assisting the home care or hospice team in achieving patient goals.

The Care Guidelines, or topics, are organized alphabetically for easy retrieval and review of needed information. Keep in mind that there may be more than one Care Guideline that is applicable to your patient. For example, when caring for a hospice patient with cancer, refer to both "Hospice Care" and "Cancer Care". Similarly, for the patient with diabetes mellitus with a wound, the reader is referred to both "Diabetes Mellitus Care" and "Wound Care".

1) **Definition of the Problem or Diagnosis:** This section contains a brief description or definition of the diagnosis or care problem that is addressed in the specific Care Guideline. These definitions may include a medical diagnosis, such as amputation, or a nursing diagnosis, such as pain and describe the problem in practical terms.

2) **General Information:** This section contains general information on a particular patient problem gathered from experience, practice, and education. This information assists the HHA in safely caring for the patient.

3) **Home Health Aide Goals for Care:** These goals are specific to the functions of the HHA and are brief statements that are based on the patient problem and diagnosis. As home care moves to a more outcome-based practice, the HHA goals support the entire team's efforts of working together to achieve pre-determined, patient-centered outcomes or measurable

goals of care. "Other goals" are listed as the last goal under Goals of Care so the team may assist the HHA in identifying additional goals that are based on a patient's unique needs and situation.

4) **Personal Care Considerations:** This section identifies areas relating to the patient's condition and lists unique personal care information that may assist the HHA in performing these tasks. For example, the ideal time for skin inspection and identification of any skin changes is during the patient's bath. Any changed personal care considerations that should be reported to the supervisor can then be integrated into the aide care plan for improving patient care and team communication.

5) **Safety Considerations:** Because safety considerations are such an integral part of safe and effective home care, this section describes specific actions or information that the HHA can use for early identification or prevention of some problems. Any problems identified should be communicated to the supervisor.

6) **Documentation Tips:** These instructions are the basis for meeting the standards and requirements of effective home care documentation. For an in depth discussion about documentation, please refer to Chapter Five.

7) **Special Considerations:** This section seeks to provide important information that does not specifically fit into the above mentioned categories. Examples include nutrition or dietary needs, based on the Care Guideline discussed. This section also has blank lines to allow the HHA to document additional considerations for a particular patient problem or a special patient program. The information may be provided by

the aide coordinator or supervisor. This individualization of care practices encourages the identification and sharing of patient information among home care team members. Additional lines are added in this section to allow for individualization or for your organization's special instruction(s).

____

____

____

PART ONE

HOME HEALTH AIDE: A VERY IMPORTANT ROLE

CHAPTER ONE

THE HOME HEALTH AIDE: OVERVIEW OF A VERY IMPORTANT ROLE

Most people who have ever been inpatients in a hospital will probably say they could not wait to go home. Home is a comfortable place where people can make their own decisions, eat familiar foods, and get better with the assistance of family, friends, and even pets. Have you thought about what you would do if you were ill and needed more assistance and you had no one to help? Your home health or hospice employer provides health care-related services to meet the unique needs of patients in just such a situation.

The need for qualified and competent home health aides (HHA) is expected to grow dramatically in the coming decade. According to a report from the U.S. Bureau of Labor Statistics, aides account for 27% of home care jobs. In another report from the same agency, aides and physician assistants are the two fastest growing health care occupations with aides leading the way. There is also the belief that the role of the aide will expand as additional duties and responsibilities are required to provide health care services to the growing home care marketplace.

THE VALUED ROLE OF THE HOME HEALTH AIDE - MORE IMPORTANT THAN EVER!

The role of the aide is important for many reasons. It is often the care provided by the aide that enables patients to stay at home, surrounded by their support systems. The home care program or hospice organization depends on the aide to provide gentle support, assistance with activities of daily living (ADLs), as well as care for sick and dying patients.

One of the unique aspects of personal care is that even though home health aides and patients have just met, aides have access to their patients' most personal belonging – their bodies. All personal care workers must remember that they are guests in their patients' home and must always be respectful of the patient's privacy, personal belongings, and most importantly, patient and family confidentiality.

We all have heard about the problem of the increased cost of health care. Most health insurance plans include payment for all or part of home care or hospice services. In an effort to control costs, some insurance companies or managed care organizations decide how long and how much care a patient may receive.

In most cases, in order for the service to be covered by a health insurance plan, the patient's doctor must write an "order". This "order" is similar to a prescription, covering the specific services needed by the patient. The first visit to the patient's home is usually done by a registered nurse or therapist. This clinician assesses the patient and then discusses the identified patient needs with the patient, family, and physician. Then the home care team members decide how to best meet those needs. For those patients cared for at home through "hospice" there is also a specialized team. A plan of care is created, including medications, treatments, and services to be carried out by each team member. Nursing (RN), physical therapy (PT), occupational therapy (OT), speech language pathology therapy (SLP), medical social services (MSS), and other types of services and/or visits may vary and last about thirty to forty-five minutes or longer, based on the patient's needs. Home health aide visits also vary in length of time based on the patient's identified needs. For example, a visit may extend one to three hours or more, depending upon how independent patients are in caring for themselves. Some patients need more hours of care and aides may be there for "shifts".

There are unique and challenging roles as an HHA. You may be the first line of defense - - to observe a change in your patient that must be reported to the nurse supervisor! Role variation may differ with the focus or mission statement of the program. The older adult community, sick or frail children, young adults stricken with disabling or chronic diseases, and other special patient populations are within the scope of the modern HHAs role. Differences in patient populations allow the career HHA to develop his/her specialty interest areas.

ABOUT YOU

You have been specially chosen by your organization because of your skills and training. Your references, skills, and qualifications provided the basis for your joining the home care or hospice organization's team. Congratulations and welcome to the growing and exciting world of home care! Now that you are a team member, let's explore the qualities that are very important for you to nurture and maintain in home care.

THE REQUIREMENTS AND QUALITIES NEEDED TO BE A SUCCESSFUL HOME HEALTH AIDE

The following competencies are basic to a successful career as a HHA:

Interpersonal Communication Skills
- Present a neat and professional appearance

- Follow directions accurately
- Use effective listening skills
- Communicate clearly and positively with patients, families, team members, and others

Reporting Skills
- Notify supervisor of any change in the patient's condition (immediately, depending on the situation)
- Maintain up-to-date records regarding your health (e.g., TB test, others)
- Create and submit legible and timely documentation
- Understand and comply with the policies and procedures of the organization

Clinical Caregiving Skills
- Attend and pass home health aide training program –certified home health aide, by the state, or other specialty training
- Complete competency evaluation with skills demonstration
- Attend required continuing education programs and appropriate staff meetings

Safety Skills
- Pay attention to detail for personal and patient home environment safety skills
- Practice effective infection control
- Possess a safe driving record and have reliable transportation
- Have the ability to navigate and use transportation options

Personal Skills
- Possess a caring and kind manner toward people
- Respect patients' individual lifestyles, choices, and beliefs
- Maintain patient confidentiality
- Participate in coordination of care between team members

- Have a positive attitude and good sense of humor
- Be flexible
- Possess high integrity and ethical behavior
  (do the "right thing")

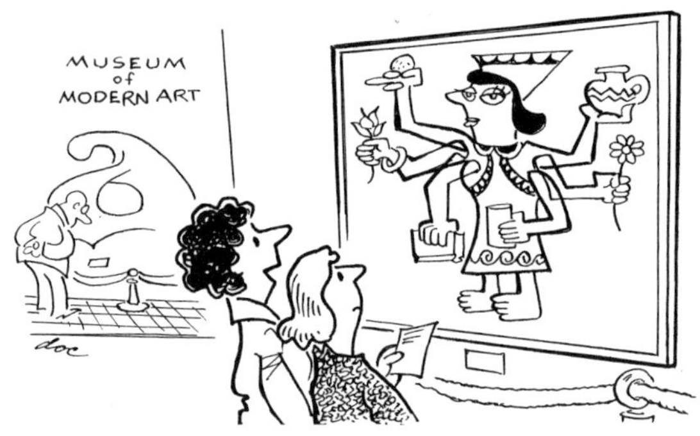

"SHE WOULD BE A GREAT HOME HEALTH AIDE."

THE SKILLS NEEDED TO BE A SUCCESSFUL HOME HEALTH AIDE

The objective of the home health aide is to provide personal care to patients while promoting home environment safety and support according to the organization's policies and procedures. The HHA role is vital in assisting patients to achieve their optimal level of independence and self-care when possible. This list is not all inclusive. Actual duties, tasks, and assignments are based on the patient's individualized plan of care (POC) needs as well as the organization's mission and applicable federal, state, and local regulations or laws.

As directed by the plan of care:

Assists Patients with Personal Care
- Personal hygiene care
- Bathing
- Hair, skin, and fingernail care

- Shaving (for male patients)
- Mouth and oral hygiene care
- Catheter care
- Peri-care
- Foot care (but does **not** cut toenails)
- Ear care
- Toileting assistance including commodes, bedpans, and urinals
- Vital signs (T-P-R (temperature, pulse, respirations), blood pressure, pain)
- Grooming and dressing
- Nutritious meal preparation per prescribed diet
- Plans meals and shops for food as directed by supervisor
- Assists with enemas, catheter care, and colostomy care (if organization allows)
- Simple dressing as directed by nurse supervisor
- Assists with **self-administration of medications**

Assist Patients with Ambulation and Exercise
- Assistance with walker, quad cane, other assistive devices
- ADL (Activities of Daily Living) training
- Ambulation
- Range of motion and home exercise program as directed by the therapist or nurse
- Bedbound care (including frequent changes in body position)
- Proper use and safety of mechanical lift
- Effective body mechanics while providing care
- Safe lifting and transferring of patients
- Use and care of prosthetics or orthotics for functional positioning
- Teaching families, role modeling for independence in ADLs and for preparation for discharge, and "self-care" planning
- Application/assistance with elastic stockings

Maintain Healthful and Safe Environment

- Reports unsafe conditions in the home
- Cleans patient care area
- Provides light housekeeping duties related to patient care
- Promotes home environment safety while providing care
- Assists with **self-administered medications**
- Complies with organization's policies and procedures related to safety, security, and disaster preparedness
- Always perform duties in compliance with state regulations, Medicare, the organization policies and procedures, and with competency and other required training

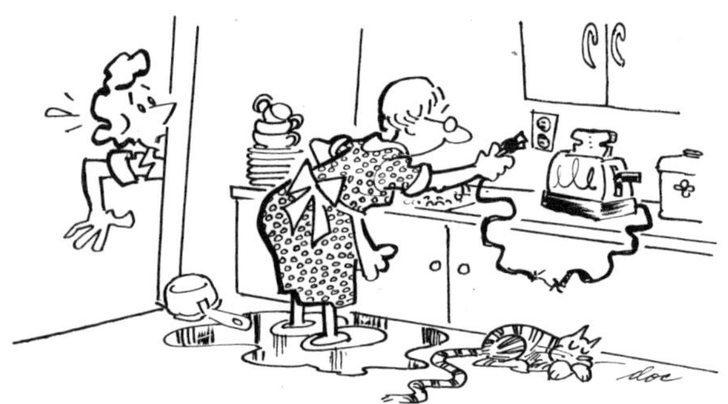

Promotes Infection Control Standards

- Washes hands effectively
- Properly and appropriately utilizes personal protection equipment (PPE) while providing care as needed (i.e. gloves, gowns, aprons,masks, eye shields)
- Wears plastic apron when providing direct care
- Wears gloves while providing any personal care
- Practices standard precautions/follows organzation's infection control policeies at all times
- Properly disposes of bodily fluids
- Performs household tasks as needed with consideration of infection control

- Follows agency/organizational infection
  control policies

Displays Caring Behavior
- Practices comfort measures (e.g., massage, positioning
  or turning)
- Cares for patients sensitively at end-of-life
- Demonstrates customer service behaviors (e.g.,
  anticipates needs before being asked)
- Considers and respects patient preferences
- Recognizes needs and rights of patients
- Monitors for abuse and/or neglect and immediately
  reports to supervisor
- Supports patient to return to best level of functioning
- Always explains procedures before performing them
- Respects patient's privacy (HIPAA)
- Maintains confidentiality at all times
- Is polite in interactions with patients, family members,
  and peers
- Recognizes and demonstrates respect for
  cultural diversity

Documents Patient Care
- Writes clearly and legibly
- Submits timely documentation
- Completes records accurately
- Submits appropriate completed records

Reports to Supervisor
- Reports changes in patient's conditions or needs
- Shows sound judgment
- Makes recommendations for improving patient care
- Reports to supervisor as required in a timely manner
- Reports requests from patient such as scheduling
  changes

Demonstrates Responsibility for Self-Development
- Identifies areas needed for improving knowledge
- Participates in organizational staff meetings

- Presents a professional and positive image
- Represents the organization as a reflection of its mission
- Promotes/participates in quality improvement as related to organizational studies/initiatives

Others: (Fill in based on organizational or supervisor's requirements)

____

____

____

____

____

ORIENTATION: AN IMPORTANT TIME

The importance of an effective orientation cannot be overstated. The orientation period is the time to ask questions, become comfortable with your new peer group, and receive any needed education and information to assist you in being a dedicated and competent home health aide. This orientation period is also the time to ask any questions about documentation, patient care, or other concerns.

Some programs have the new home health aide accompanied by a nurse or experienced "senior" aide on the initial visits. This "buddy" system gives the new aide a role model or mentor to assist in the transition to a new organization. Some programs supervise each aide every two weeks, a homemaker once a month, and others more often, based on the patient's unique needs, contractual arrangements, and regulations. These "joint visits" with the supervisor also clarify for patients and their families the role the aide will play in caregiving. The intent is that this will prevent family members or clients from asking the aide to provide care that is inappropriate, unsafe, or outside of the aide's responsibilities. This time is also helpful to the nursing supervisor to gather information regarding performance evaluations.

Though you believe the supervisor may be busy, if there is a question at any time about patient care, documentation, or scheduling problems, arrange a time to talk or meet with your supervisor. Remember, the goal of orientation is to assure that each aide receives both general and specific information to enable safe and effective performance of duties required for the patient, and assigned by the supervising team member. Think of orientation as a time to learn all that there is to become a better home health aide!

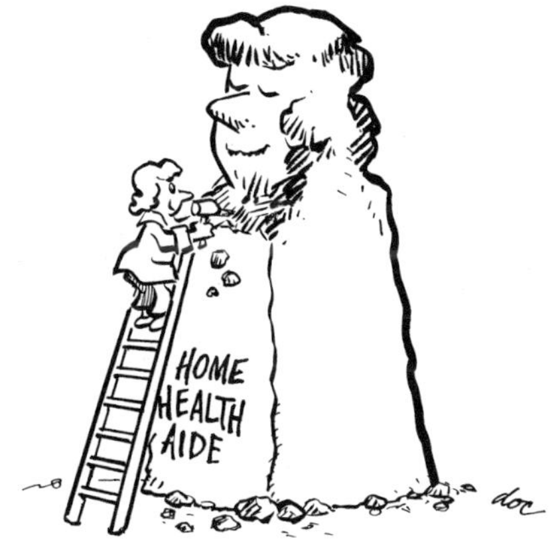

HIGHLIGHTS OF AN
EFFECTIVE ORIENTATION

Though there are differences between agencies and organizations regarding aide orientation, the following details some highlights of an effective orientation:

Organizational Information

- Welcome to the organization
- Mission statement
- Organizational chart
- Introduction to home care
- Program philosophy and scope of services
- Human resources and personnel policies unique to the agency

  (This can include reviewing and signing your job description and completing required paperwork)

- Administrative information (e.g. time cards, mileage, parking, paydays, scheduling, etc.)
- Confidentiality, patient bill of rights and responsibilities, and other policies unique to the program
- Agency policies and procedures
- Dress code or uniform policies
- Reporting requirements
- Communication skills, agency communication systems, and lines of communication
- How to ask for time off, who to call if ill
- Obtaining supplies, gloves, gowns, etc.
- Any continuing education requirements (exams, etc.) to demonstrate competency
- Role of payer regulations, etc.

Caregiving Role Information

- Important role of the home health aide or hospice aide
- Roles of the individual disciplines or careteam members (OT, PT, others)
- Personal care services, hygiene, standard precautions
- Principles of effective nutrition and meal planning
- Safety in home care (e.g. body mechanics, lumbar support belts, car and personal)
- Patient care forms and documentation (record keeping and reporting)

- Human life cycles and the impact of illness or disability
- Importance of self-care activities
- Courtesy and customer service and interpersonal relations
- First aid and emergency guidelines
- Responsibilities when there is a disruption in care due to disaster/ emergency/ weather
- Reporting of patient status changes
- Identifying and reporting potential victims of abuse /neglect
- Skill review and demonstration
- Agency/organization performance improvement projects
- Homebound criteria for Medicare and other rules and regulations

Other Information
- Hospice, pediatric, psychiatric, rehabilitation, maternity, geriatric, and other specialty program information
- Map reading skills

   Others: (Fill in based on supervisor's requirements)

____

____

____

WORKING WITHIN THE SCOPE
OF THE POSITION DESCRIPTION

   The orientation period is also the time new aides are informed of tasks and duties that they may or may not perform within the scope of their position description. There are state laws that affect certified, licensed, and unlicensed personnel, such as the aide. For example, by law, administering medications and changing dressings are usually not within the scope of what the home health aide can do. It is for this reason that aides must understand clearly their position description and when to ask or call the licensed nurse for direction. In addition, state laws vary, and as such, **aides should ask their supervisor before performing any task that is not understood or has not been previously performed.** Your employer may have copies of the applicable state law for your review and information.

The goal of home care is to provide safe and effective care to patients in their homes. If it appears that there is an unsafe situation or that a patient is receiving ineffective care, notify the aide supervisor or other appropriate manager.

SUMMARY

By the end of an effective orientation process, the aide should be able to:

- Establish and maintain a relationship with the agency supervisor.
- Understand and adhere to the patient activities specified on the aide plan of care.
- Perform the patient care tasks, activities, and other responsibilities as stated in the aide position description.
- Understand the expectations the organization has of the aide role.
- Know who to call at the organization for questions relating to patient care and administrative or other concerns.
- Know who your first patients are and make sure you have directions to their homes!

REVIEW EXERCISES

1) List three team members who may be involved in the plan of care. (See page 3).
2) Identify five of the qualities needed to be a successful home health aide. (See page 4, 5, 6).
3) Describe two reasons why the orientation period is an important time for the aide. (See page 10-11).
4) State five highlights of an effective orientation program. (See pages 11, 12, 13).
5) Write a one or two paragraph answer to the following question: "Why I would make a very good home health aide."

CHAPTER TWO

THE SPECIAL AND VALUED SKILLS NEEDED IN HOME CARE

The Home Health Aide possesses special skills related to:

- Determining how well patients can manage on their own;
- Observing patient behaviors with friends,family, and other health care team members;
- Noting the patient's improvement in functional self-care behaviors and independence; and
- Noting the patient's compliance (adherence)to care regimens and behaviors.

Home care team members should do their best to do things in the way the patient prefers. For example, some people prefer to brush their teeth before eating, and others, after they eat. Many patients have specific foods they like to eat at certain meals, even though that may seem strange or different to you. Some patients do not feel the need to bathe everyday. Others may allow their pets in areas of the home where you would not. Appreciating the similarities as well as the differences among all people is an important part of being an effective home health aide.

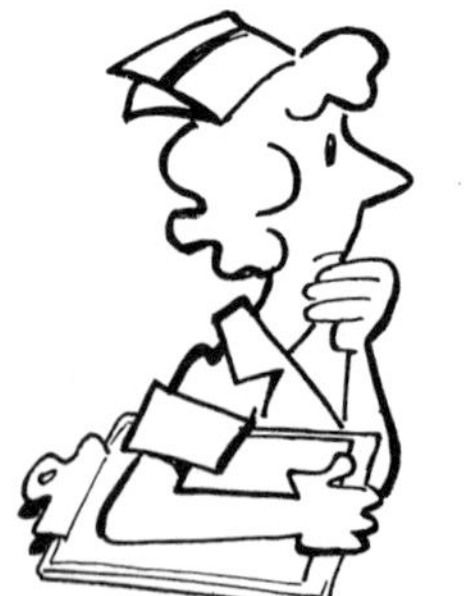
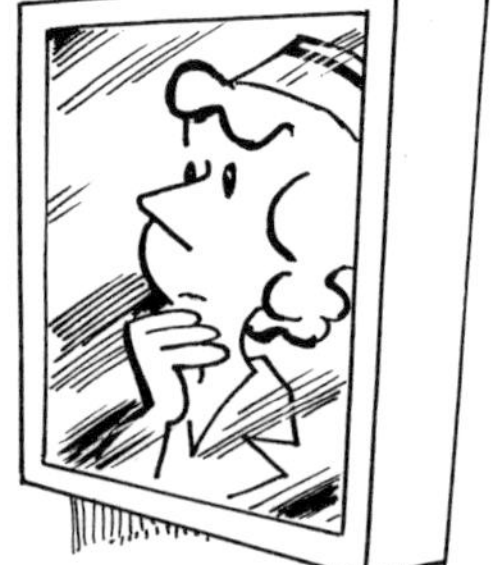

INTERPERSONAL QUALITIES

Home health aides have a lot of important information to remember. Interpersonal qualities and communication with staff and patients are as important as personal caregiving skills. Communication with staff and patients must be courteous and relayed in a way that is clearly understood. We know how we would like our own family member to be treated by a HHA, and that is the way we always should treat all patients.

Personal characteristics that patients and families seek in home health aides are:

- Compatibility
- Reliability
- Promptness
- Capability
- Trustworthiness and honesty
- Ability to be understood
- Patience, caring, and kindness
- Courtesy
- Promotion of independence
- Ability to listen
- Confidence in the ability to do the best job possible
- Clean and neat professional appearance

Compatibility means that you and the patient can get along. Home health care often involves meeting new people, many of whom you would not choose for a friend, but who still need your help. Personality "fit" is important because part of home health care involves helping patients gain independence. For this to happen, it is important that patients develop a trusting relationship with their home health care team members.

During the visit, conversation with patients is as necessary as physical care. There may be times when the patient and aide do not agree, and certain subjects should be avoided. This is the time to remember that we are a guest in the patient's home and the patient, as a customer, is "always right". If aides feel as though these disagreements interfere with their ability to care for the patient properly, they should talk to the supervisor or primary nurse about the problem. Occasionally, the aide may have an assignment change, and that should not be viewed as negative. Someone else may possess different skills that simply make a better match with the patient. When personalities conflict, this may inhibit the development and progression of wellness that comes with an effective therapeutic relationship. Try not to label patients who may have difficulty getting along with their caregivers, there may be a reason for their negative behavior. Remember, home care patients may have serious health problems that affect their behavior. Many times their environment and personal health are the only things they can control.

Reliability means that a person completes all assigned responsibilities. One sick call can disrupt patients' as well as other home health aides' schedules. Two sick calls may disrupt twelve patients and up to twelve more aides. Certainly when one is ill, a sick call is appropriate for the aides' and patients' benefit, but if you "just don't feel like working", think again. The role of being an aide is too important to be taken lightly. Other people are counting on you! The aide is the center of many patients' lives during their recovery. A substitute aide can be compared to a substitute teacher, he or she can do the job, but it won't be the same.

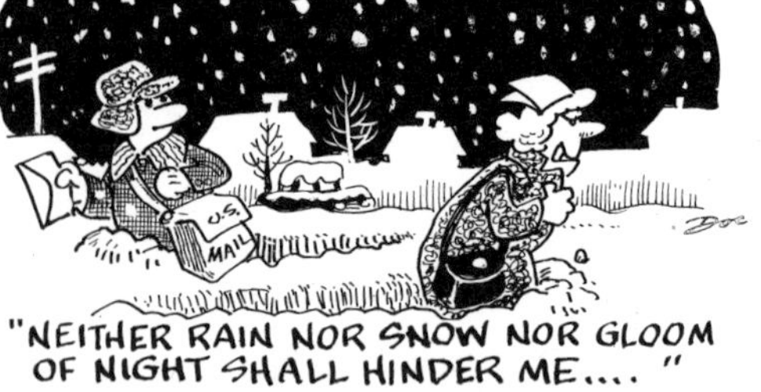

Promptness is a must to keep organized, ensure patient satisfaction, and to meet your supervisor's expectations. All home care staff must allow for traveling time between patients. The amount of time this will take is dependent upon distances, traffic patterns, parking, or public transportation. Aides should notify the scheduling staff if the time allowed is not enough. Caregivers, including family members, who meet other needs of the patient, depend upon the aide consistently to be on time. This is especially true with those patients who cannot be left alone.

Capability means accurately performing all the necessary tasks on the patient's care plan. Most patients' care involves routine tasks with which the aide is familiar. Whenever you come across a procedure or duty that is part of the care plan and of which you are unsure (not comfortable or unfamiliar with), you must immediately make this known to your supervisor. The nurse will demonstrate or teach you the new task, such as using a Hoyer lift or measuring and emptying drainage bags and recording the proper amount. **Never** perform a procedure without being taught how to do it first.

Aides are from a variety of backgrounds, and may be less familiar with specific products and their uses. All personal, cosmetic, or cleaning products to be used with patient care should be identified during the introduction to the patient, by the nurse or therapist, to ensure patient safety.

You may be asked by your supervisor to demonstrate a specific task to determine your competency. This may bolster your comfort level as well as your patient's during the procedure. This is to assure the safety of the staff and the patient. Always tell your supervisor when you are unfamiliar with a procedure you are asked to do.

Trustworthiness and honesty is a mandatory quality of all home care staff. The aide may see items or hear conversations that must be kept private and confidential. Staff who are given a key to a home must be very careful to keep it safe. While putting away clothing, the aide may observe money or jewelry, hidden or not, which also must be kept confidential. However, large amounts of money should be reported to your supervisor to be secured, especially if the patient's or caregiver's mental status is in question, or if there are many providers involved in the case.

The ability to be understood by the patient is essential. Communication is a major aspect of all home health care. Some aide certification courses have English/Spanish as a second language as part of the classroom work. To be sure they can be understood by their patients, aides should practice any specific words they find difficult to pronounce. Many patients have some form of hearing loss, and speaking clearly and slowly and in a low pitch/tone helps the patient understand. Speaking louder may not help and may even be more confusing to the patient.

Patients may have problems with communication. Some patients who have had strokes, also called cerebral vascular accidents or CVAs, cannot understand what is said to them due to brain damage. Other CVAs can cause speech difficulty that ranges from mild impediments to loss of speech. The orientation visit assessment should include a reference to any specific communication needs of the new patient and how those needs should be met by the caregiver team.

Aides who speak fluent English and another language can be valuable resources to the organization. Aides who are bilingual can take care of patients who speak other languages thus offering their organization the flexibility to care for a wider range of patients. Remember, communication in any language only occurs when both parties can be understood.

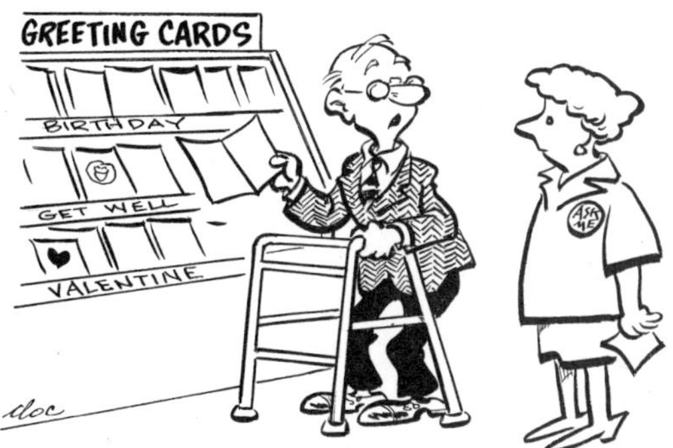

"DON'T YOU HAVE A SPECIAL VALENTINE DAY CARD FOR A HOME HEALTH AIDE?"

Patience, caring, and kindness are also necessary characteristics for all health care workers. Patience is watching patients slowly button a shirt, even when you could do it for them in half the time. You watch because you know it important for them to keep doing whatever they can for themselves. Caring can be shown in many ways:

- Fluffing a pillow
- Sensing the patient is upset by a change in his/her voice or tearing
- Making sure the patient's cane or walker is nearby
- Placing a glass of water and the phone nearby and within easy reach before leaving
- Making sure windows are open or closed (depending on the weather, the patient's choice, and home safety considerations)
- Assisting in keeping the patient oriented to time, place, family, local and national events through discussion, reading the paper, and turning on news on the radio or television
- Wearing a smile when you enter, as you care for the patient, and when you leave each day

Courtesy and being respectful are worthy human, as well as professional, behaviors. In addition, it is part of the Patient Bill of Rights that patients have a right to participate in planning their care. When we are performing tasks for patients, it is important to remember that they used to do everything for and perhaps by themselves. Patients are happier if we perform these duties the way patients would do them themselves, if they could. For example, when feeding patients, ask if they prefer to eat all the vegetables first or do they like to have a little of each part of the meal at a time. A patient may prefer to have the top sheet not tucked in. Courtesy and respect involve asking how they would like things done, not assuming our way of doing things is the only way. Another example of courtesy is asking patients what you should call them, e.g., "Mrs. Smith" or "Molly". Courtesy is asking permission to use the phone.

Promotion of Independence is always a primary goal of care. Even if the only task patients can perform independently is washing their face, that ability should be encouraged. Once in a while, patients may ask the aide to do something that they can do for themselves. The aide must gently persuade the patient to continue performing any tasks they can safely do themselves.

The aide should ask the nurse or therapist at the patient introduction how much they should do for the patient. Then as aides observe the patient's increased strength and independence, they can begin to do less for the patient. Aides should be informed by the nurse or therapist as patient discharge approaches that the patient must assume more and more of his or her care. Encourage the patient to do as much as possible as he/she can safely do for himself/herself. This is to prevent the patient from becoming too dependent on the aide and then suddenly losing the aide due to discharge from the home health care organization.

Remember, we are not being fair to patients when we do for them what they can still safely do for them-

**selves. The aide needs to foster and support independ-
ence, not dependence, on the home care staff.**

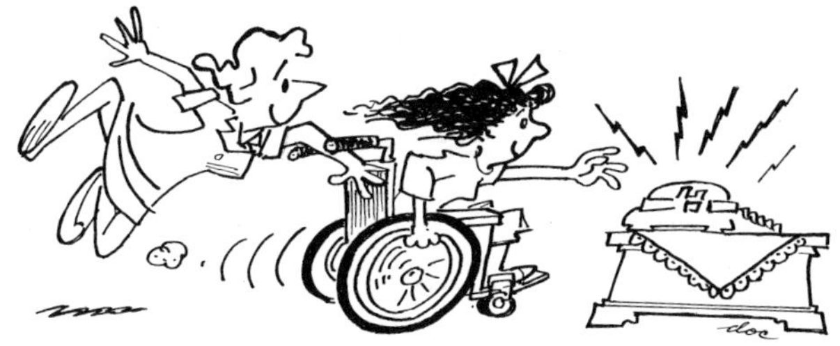

However, if the patient is too sick, tired, or generally refuses, we still must provide compassionate care and services to our patient. For some patients, involving them in their care may mean allowing them to choose their clothing or breakfast foods. Even the most dependent patients may want to make small choices in their everyday schedule, and that should be allowed and encouraged. The patients' ability to participate in their care planning improves their feelings of self-worth and control. This is true both in cases of chronic care and for those patients nearing discharge after successful rehabilitation.

The ability to listen is a skill we all have to work on regularly. Because home care is a people business, it is very much about listening to the needs of our patients and their families and friends. Home health care is all about listening and becoming aware of:

- Changes in mental status
- Changes in voice strength
- Changes in emotions
- Changes in caregiver or community support
- Changes in language – elders who have English as a second language (ESL) and have been speaking English may revert to their original language
- The meaning in and behind the words and body communications

There will be times when the aide will just listen and not speak. Often patients live alone and there may be days when the aide is the only person the patient has to talk to, and with. In these situations, just listening may be valued immeasurably by the patient. Many times the aide is the patient's connection to the outside world. However, do not provide the patient or caregiver with your home phone or cell phone number.

Patients may make gestures that do not match what they are saying, or they may roll their eyes when speaking to family members. These actions are called nonverbal communication or body language. Sometimes nonverbal communication strengthens what patients are saying and other times it seems to show the opposite of what they are verbally expressing.

The aide's sensitivity to patients' individual personalities through the ability to adjust to changes brought on by illness or wellness will help the aide improve communication skills. Your supervisor can assist you with patients who have communication problems or identify translators for patients with language barriers.

Confidence in ability to do the best job possible includes continually developing the skills you need to have to perform your job. Confidence comes from doing your job well and knowing you have the information, training, and support needed to do your job. You have the power to increase your confidence through:

- Ongoing education and training programs
- Inservice education opportunities
- Obtaining feedback from your supervisor and patients (some questions to ask include: "What can I do better?" and "How can I help?")

The above points can serve as the basis for your own continuous quality improvement process and improving your skills as a home health aide.

Clean and neat professional appearance is a hallmark of a successful home health aide. Your neat appearance demonstrates to others that you care about yourself, that you strive to do your best for your patients and your organization. As a team member, it is your responsibility to be neat and clean, and in uniform as defined by your organization's policy. This includes not smoking and not using any perfumes that could irritate already sick patients and always wearing your identification badge.

For a discussion on "Dressing for success in home care", see Chapter Nine, "Administrative Responsibilities".

REPORTING CHANGES IN PATIENT STATUS

The aide's observing, identifying and reporting changes in patient status is one of their most important roles. Find out from your supervisor how you should communicate patient changes. Sometimes your observations should be checked by the nurse or therapist right away. For this reason, you should know how to reach the nurse, therapist, and your supervisor immediately. Following the aide care plan is crucial. If the patient needs have changed you must contact the nurse immediately so revision of the aide care plan can occur.

The patient may tell you specifically not to tell the nurse about something that you think you should report. (Patients tell nurses not to call their doctors, too!) The nurse must be told about changes for which you have been asked to watch. In these cases, speak to the nurse at the office rather than call from the patient's home unless you think it is an emergency. If you have a cell phone, you may have to step outside to call your supervisor. Because you are in the patient's home, you may not use the phone without the patient's permission. Should you decide to call the nurse from your next visit, remember you may only do so if you can speak privately.

Coordination of care involves reporting issues in a timely manner. Examples of patient care events that must be reported to your supervisor are:

- Changes in breathing
- Skin breakdown or red or pink areas
- Changes in eating habits
- Changes in bowel/urine output
- Falls (witnessed and unwitnessed)
- Bleeding, bruising
- Redness, swelling in any location
- Fever
- Increased shortness of breath, coughing, or respiratory rate
- Pain, sudden onset or worsening
- Changes in patient's level of alertness or orientation
- Death in the patient's family
- Any verbal/physical abuse of patient or aide
- Safety concerns regarding the patient or aide
- Swelling of extremities
- Not taking medication according to schedule
- Patient complaints (e.g. "racing heartbeat", chest pain, etc.)
- Profuse sweating
- Lack of food, heat, liquids, or money to cover these items
- Lack of necessary items for care: clean linen, clothing, blankets, toilet articles
- Changes in ambulation, toileting activities
- Knowledge of the patient regularly or frequently leaving the home (if the patient is required to be homebound by Medicare)
- Mental changes such as agitation, confusion, not "making sense" in a usually clear and alert patient, anger, aggression, etc.
- Changes in caregiver status

- When you believe the patient needs to be seen by the doctor/ the nurse due to a worsening of condition
- Changes in weight
- Signs of low blood sugar
- Change in vital signs (high temperature, elevated/drop in blood pressure, pulse irregular, increase in pain)
- Any other change, difference, or other information that affects your patient including signs of possible abuse, neglect, or exploitation
- An ambulance is at the patient's home or has been there since your last visit.
- Your patient dies or died since your last visit and you and/or the agency/employer were not notified of the patient's passing.
- Always document on your note who, why, and what you reported. This includes name of the person you reported the problem to, when you reported, and what specifically you reported about the patient.
- **When in doubt - - call your supervisor.**

SUMMARY

Successful home health aides have important interpersonal qualities that contribute to their effectiveness. These skills help the aide and the patients forge a working relationship needed to help the patient meet program goals. This interpersonal relationship helps the aide work with family members and identify changes in their patients' status, which then must be reported to the supervisor. The demonstration of good communication skills every day with your peers and supervisor, as well as with patients and their families, also contributes to your organization's patient satisfaction. Because home care is a "people" business, communication is a very important part of the aide's job.

REVIEW EXERCISES

1) List four of the interpersonal qualities that are positive characteristics that patients and families want in aides. Explain the meaning of each characteristic. (See page 17).
2) Explain why "we are not being fair to patients when we do for them what they can still do for themselves". (See page 22-23).
3) Describe why the skill of listening is so important in home care. (See page 23-24).
4) State the procedure for contacting your supervisor to communicate patient changes.
5) Name ten examples of patient care events or changes that must be reported to your supervisor. (See page 26-27).

CHAPTER THREE

KEY COMPONENTS
OF HOME CARE PRACTICE

The key components of home care practice for the aide include the Patient's Bill of Rights and Responsibilities, confidentiality, ethics, sensitivity to values and lifestyles, and patient and family involvement in care. These important components are basic to home care and hospice organizations and are further explained in subsequent chapters, where noted. Questions and topics needing additional clarification or more information should be taken to the supervisor.

PATIENT BILL OF RIGHTS
AND RESPONSIBILITIES

All patients cared for by hospitals, home care, and hospice organizations are entitled to exercise their rights as outlined in the Patient Bill of Rights and Responsibilities. The home care or hospice organization must protect and promote the exercise or use of these rights. These patient rights include the expectation that home care and hospice team members respect patient wishes, privacy, values, and are careful with patient furnishings and property. It is easier to understand these important concepts if aides think of themselves as guests in their patients' homes. In other words, if you were the patient, how would you expect to be treated?

Prior to providing care, the admitting nurse or therapist must inform the patients and family caregivers of their rights. By reviewing the Patient Bill of Rights and Responsibilities, the patient knows, and has in writing, what to expect from the home care or hospice organization. Usually, the patient and family caregivers sign and receive a copy the Patient Bill of Rights. This enables them to refer to this information as needed. The Patient Bill of Rights and Responsibilities should be familiar to all home care staff as many organizations include this information in their general or comprehensive orientation. If this information was not provided at orientation, consider requesting a copy from your supervisor. The following is a general list and your organization's Bill of Rights may look different.

PATIENT BILL OF RIGHTS AND RESPONSIBILITIES

I.   Right to have medical and personal information held in confidence by all members of the health care team

II.   Right to refuse to participate in care, even after hearing about the consequences of refusing that care.

III.   Right to choose their doctor.

IV.   Right to participate in planning their care.

V.   Right to quality medical and home healthcare delivered by a trained and competent staff.

VI.   Right to be informed about services offered and the cost for services before services are provided.

VII.   Right to respect, dignity, and consideration of their individuality.

VIII.   Right to be fully informed about changes in service delivery.

IX.   Right to a prompt response to questions about their care, consequences of refusal of care, and to questions about information contained in their home health care record.

CONFIDENTIALITY

Aides must share patient information with other home care team members in order to meet the patient's unique care needs. Sharing patient information brings up the important issue of confidentiality. Confidentiality in home care means that patients are not discussed except 1) with the aide supervisor and 2) other care team members who are involved with the care of your patient. Information you hear or learn from patients, their family or friends should not be discussed outside of their home, unless it is clearly related to the patient's safety and care. Your supervisor is the best judge in this situation.

PRIVACY AND HIPAA

The term HIPAA is used frequently in health care. The U.S. government was called on to issue patient privacy protections as part of the Health Insurance Portability and Accountability Act (HIPAA) of 1996. HIPAA included rules designed to encourage health care providers such as home care, hospice, hospitals and other health care organizations to provide electronic transactions. The HIPAA also required safeguards to protect the security and confidentiality of health information. Simply put, the regulations protect medical records and other individually identifiable health information, whether it is on paper, in computers, or communicated orally. Some of the key provisions of these standards include: access to medical records/information, notice of privacy practice where patients are provided a notice which informs of their rights under the privacy regulation. You may have experienced this when you are asked to sign or initial or otherwise acknowledge that you received this notice when you go to your doctor's office.

All of these examples are provisions of the HIPAA. Ask your supervisor if you have any questions about HIPAA and your organization.

ETHICS IN HOME CARE

Ethics is a term that is used in health care practice. What are ethics? Ethics concern moral issues, choices, or dilemmas, that may make the aide and others involved in patient care feel uncomfortable. Common examples of ethical dilemmas include:

1) When the family disagrees about what is "best" for the patient,
2) When the family doesn't want the patient to go to a nursing home or other setting, even when in the opinion of the health care team that may be better for the patient,
3) When you believe a patient is being neglected, exploited, or abused and the family pretends that everything is okay,
4) When a patient with chronic lung disease, who has been admitted to the hospital more than once for pneumonia, continues to smoke against the doctor's orders,
5) When patients with diabetes drink alcoholic beverages and "forget" their daily insulin, and, when it is time to eat, only want chocolate,
6) When there is drug activity or other indications of unlawful activity.

Ethical situations such as these are as unique as the home care caseload. These situations can be very frustrating for the home care team as they try to care for their patients and do "what is best" and "the right thing". Many organizations have ethics committees or other mechanisms to address these difficult and oftentimes, frustrating and distressing patient scenarios. Moral dilemmas in home care present some of the greatest challenges in home care practice. Any of these kinds of problems should be addressed with your supervisor for safety and patient care reasons.

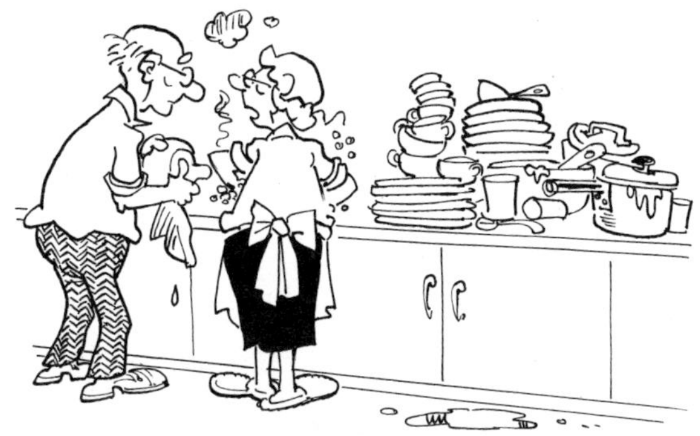

SENSITIVITY TO VALUES AND LIFESTYLES

The ethical discussion as well as the above discussion about patient rights and responsibilities leads to the topic of the patient's individual lifestyle choices. All of the things that we as individuals cherish or feel are important are called values. All people have values that must be respected, and in health care this respect must also include values with which health care team members may not always agree.

Values of patients might include:
- Religious or spiritual beliefs
- Choice of holiday celebrations
- Lifestyle choices (remaining single or choosing not to have children)

- Sexuality orientation and/or preference
- Cultural behaviors
- Attitudes toward people who seem different
- Family interactions: closeness or isolation
- Political affiliations
- Personal hygiene and cleanliness
- Other belief systems

At times you may not personally agree with the patient about particular beliefs, lifestyles, or other choices. Nevertheless, health care team members must respect and honor the patient's choice and be non-judgmental. It is not the role of the aide to try and change the patient's longstanding or respected beliefs. In home care, patients from all over the world and from diverse backgrounds are provided with care. Patients and their families may have belief systems, languages, or accepted health treatments different from those usually accepted in our health culture. Respect and value must be shown to these unique cultural behaviors and habits. This sensitivity to values and lifestyles has special meaning to patients and their families during illness and recovery, and during the dying process.

These values are personal to each individual, and should be respected. However, unlawful activity, signs and symptoms of potential abuse/neglect of the patient, or neglect of the patient's needs by family or caregivers should not be accepted as personal choice and should be reported to the supervisor immediately.

PATIENT AND FAMILY INVOLVEMENT IN CARE

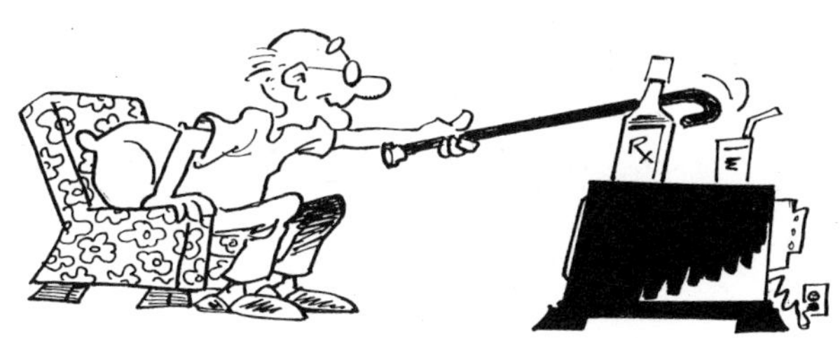

To provide individualized care, it is important that the aide ask patients how they would like things accomplished and how they would perform an activity if they could do it for themselves. This is a positive step toward treating people as individuals, given the constraints of visit time. Working with people who need home care assistance can be very gratifying. Respecting values, individuality, and the uniqueness of each human being helps us to appreciate patients and our unique differences, as well.

Sometimes it can be very difficult to stand by and watch patients do what we may believe "is not the best or correct thing". When this occurs, speak with your supervisor about the most effective way to address or cope with this feeling.

SUMMARY

The topics discussed in this chapter relate to the patient's and family's privacy and rights. We all want to live as we choose, and patients are no different. In fact, when people are sick, they may sometimes depend more on their belief systems and habits, which may be very different from our own. Respecting patients' rights and responsibilities, confidentiality, ethical issues, and sensitivity to patients' own unique lifestyles is an important part of providing quality care. By upholding these standards in home and hospice care, the aide demonstrates caring and recognizing patients' and families' needs and life patterns.

REVIEW EXERCISES

1) List three patient rights and responsibilities.
   (See page 30).
2) Describe patient confidentiality. (See page 31).
3) Identify two examples of ethical problems seen in
   home care. (See page 32).
4) Name three examples of patient values.
   (See page 33-34).
5) List 3 examples of abuse or neglect. (See page 32).
6) Explain what you would say to a family member if
   they asked you about privacy and/or HIPAA.
   (See page 31).

CHAPTER FOUR

THE TEAM CONCEPT IN HOME HEALTH CARE: WORKING TOGETHER TO HELP PATIENTS

Home health care, as well as hospice care, is unique. The care provided at home can be seen as the opposite of inpatient care, such as a nursing home or hospital, where the patients are grouped together in one setting. Your patient may be next door, 20 miles away, or even across a state or county line. Your supervisor and the other team members are not "down the hall" but a phone call away or a drive back to the office. Because of this, the importance of communicating about the patient's care needs takes on special and added importance.

Effective home health care practice supports the patient's independence and the team concept helps us all work together to help patients. We are not helping when we make patients dependent on us, especially when they need to be discharged from home health care services. In home care, it is very important to allow patients to do as much as safely possible for themselves. This can include dressing, parts of grooming or bathing, as well as other tasks.

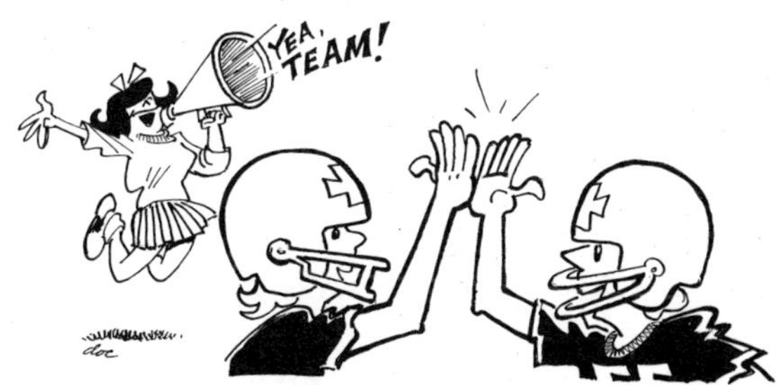

The Team Concept at Work

THE HOME HEALTH CARE TEAM

The home health care team includes the people from your program who are caring for your patient. The patient is the center of the communication among home care workers. Home care team members provide services to meet many needs of the home care patient/family.

The Home Care Team Might Include:

- Nursing = RN Registered Nurse;
  LPN/LVN = Licensed Practical/Vocational Nurse
- Physical Therapy = PT (Physical Therapist), or PTA (Physical Therapy Assistant/Aide)
- Occupational Therapy = OT (Occupational Therapist), or OTA (Occupational Therapy Assistant)
- Speech Therapy or Speech-Language Pathology = ST (Speech Therapist) or SLP (Speech-Language Pathologist)
- Medical Social Services = MSS (or MSS assistant) or Medical Social Worker (MSW)
- Home Health Aide = HHA (Be aware that HHA can also stand for home health agency.)
- Other care providers or team members may include the physician, chaplain, pharmacist, dietitian, respiratory therapist, hospice team members, volunteers, counselors, wound ostomy continence nurse (WOCN), and other specialists, based on the patient's unique needs and mission of your organization.

The Hospice Team Might Include:

- The patient and family (the unit of care in hospice)
- The Hospice Physician
- Nursing = RN Registered Nurse
- LPN/LVN =Licensed Practical/Vocational Nurse
- Social Worker/Social Work Services = SW

- Hospice Volunteers = Specially trained volunteers who work with hospice patients and their families
- Chaplain or other spiritual counselor
- Physical Therapy – PT
- Occupational Therapy –OT
- Hospice aide
- Art or music therapist

Other services and providers may vary and be based on the patient's unique hospice plan of care. They may include the massage therapist, speech therapy or speech-language pathology services, a pharmacist, a dietitian, a respiratory therapist, specialists such as wound, ostomy continence nurses (WOCN), and others, all based on the patient and program.

There may also be staff from other agencies, such as homemakers, respite workers, mental health workers, and/or meals-on-wheels representatives.

THE PLAN OF CARE

Home health care practice is driven by each patient's unique "plan of care". The plan of care or POC is created by the home health care nurse (or therapist) in conjunction with the patient's physician. This is completed after a lengthy and comprehensive initial assessment home visit. This comprehensive assessment is called "OASIS", which stands for Outcome and Assessment Information Set and is required by Medicare for most patients (your nurse is the expert on Medicare and OASIS rules). The nurse or therapist explains the rules about home care, the costs, the services offered, as well as other components of care including rights and responsibilities, privacy, and others. The POC lists the patient problems, medications, and the orders, by each team member or discipline, needed for that patient. This lengthy assessment process also in-cludes information related to HIPAA, safety issues, home care needs and emergency disaster preparedness. The POC takes into account the patient's needs and problems and is the plan that will assist the patient in meeting predetermined care goals.

Initial patient information is written on the home health aide care plan or assignment sheet. This aide assignment sheet designates specific duties to be completed during patient visits. A copy of this care plan may be left in the patient's home and be available for review by other home health care team members. As the aide becomes more familiar with the patient he/she may contribute to and help coordinate changes. When first introduced to the patient, the nurse or therapist explains specific symptoms or safety concerns to be watched for and reported should they occur. The aide can sometimes provide less care, as the patient improves, but not more. For example, a patient who at first needs to be fed may be able to feed himself as his condition improves. When changes such as these or other changes occur, call your supervisor with a report of changes in your patient's condition. The nurse or therapist may then make a new assignment. This is also called the home health aide plan of care (POC) or the aide care plan. Be aware of the importance of following the POC. Most accidents that occur to the patient or the aide happen when the care plan is not being followed.

HOME SAFETY: A MOST IMPORTANT COMPONENT OF HOME HEALTH CARE

Home safety is an example of the types of observation the nurse or therapist may address on the aide assignment sheet. For instance, the nurse may note and report to you that the patient has scatter rugs on a shiny wood floor, and this is dangerous because the patient uses a walker and may trip. This elderly patient has limited ambulatory abilities and may be prone to falls. The aide should observe the patient's ambulation and remind the patient and/or family of the need to remove or be careful when ambulating around the scatter rugs. Or, the aide may suggest that the scatter rugs be moved out of the patient's pathway. Other special observations for you to make during visits will be written directly on the care plan. Another example is if the patient declines a shower and prefers a bedbath, that is acceptable, but if a patient whose plan of care specifies bedbath wants to take a shower, this may not be done without checking with the nurse or supervisor. It is the responsibility of the home health aide to support other team member recommendations and reinforce them with their patients.

The ability of the aide to notice changes in the patient's condition or status is very important. Report those changes that the nurse or therapist requested. You should also write this information on your daily aide visit note or other forms that are used or required by your organization. In addition, the aide may see family relationships or patient behaviors which are preventing the patient from following the care plan. This information should also be reported to your supervisor.

PATIENT EXAMPLE: MR. ABLE

Mr. Able has just been discharged from St. Elsewhere General Hospital. Mr. Able's problem is swelling of his lower legs and feet due to heart failure (HF). The nurse creates a nursing plan to include such care as:

1) Check Mr. Able to make sure he is taking the medications as ordered. (This is called medication compliance.)
2) Measure the patient's ankles or other leg areas (depending on the extent of the swelling and doctor's orders).
3) Check the patient's blood pressure and vital signs every visit.
4) Assist in applying support hose if ordered
5) Daily weights since HF is Mr. Able's diagnosis and the aide care plan has this important activity listed.

The RN's corresponding goals for Mr. Able are:

1) Compliance with the new medication regimen as demonstrated by Mr. Able verbally listing the medications, the dose, and the times to the nurse
2) Decrease leg swelling demonstrated by a decrease in size of his legs since admission
3) Blood pressure within normal for patient range
4) Successful home exercise program (HEP) for Mr. Able.

Mr. Able will also have the social worker visit to address financial problems related to obtaining expensive medications. A physical therapist will visit for the purpose of increasing mobility, and developing a safe home exercise program. An occupational therapist will also visit Mr. Able for energy conservation and activities of daily living (ADL) training such as dressing or feeding himself. The occupational therapy goals are to increase his functional endurance and increase his independence in self-care with adaptive devices.

Mr. Able has five services involved in his plan of care:

1) You, the home health aide
2) The nurse, who may be called the care or case manager
3) The physical therapist,

4) Occupational therapist

5) The medical social service worker.

All of these team members need to communicate together about Mr. Able on a regular basis, making sure that Mr. Able is meeting his goals. This would include discussing whether he is recovering as planned and, if not, discussing changes to the original, agreed-upon plan. All of the team members may have input into the aide's assignment sheet or care plan, usually completed by the nurse.

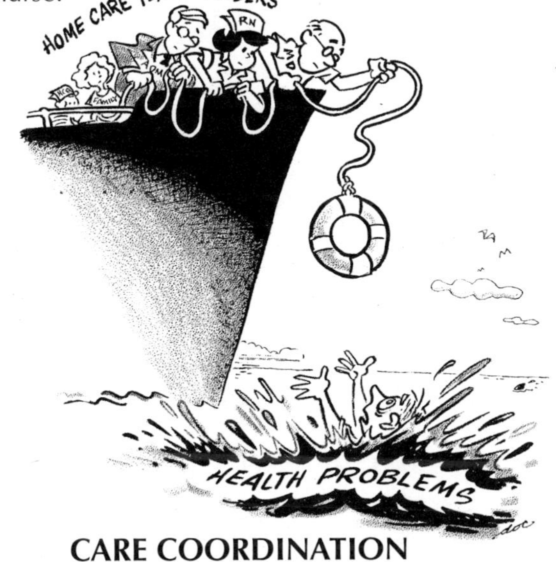

CARE COORDINATION

Care or case coordination is important for a number of reasons. There is an emphasis in health care today on being careful with limited resources and personnel. As an example, insurance companies, such as Medicare, want to be sure they are getting quality services for the amount of money they pay to agencies to provide patient care. Insurance companies also want to know that their patients are "getting better" or achieving improvement or better "outcomes" as a way to determine if they are getting their money's worth. In fact, many times the insurance company will want to see parts of the clinical record and documentation so that they can review the care for cost and quality reasons. The clinical documentation should support ongoing team communications as well as demonstrate that effective patient care is being provided. The importance of documentation, the aide's documentation specifically, is discussed in a later section of this book.

Depending upon the organization and its patients, the aide should be involved in patient care conferences and interdisciplinary meetings. Interdisciplinary means different "disciplines" or professional specialties are involved.

Some examples of care coordination include reporting changes or new pain to the nurse, notifying the physical therapist that a patient is not doing the recommended exercises, calling the supervisor to report that the patient complained of another aide not providing their bath the last time, or during a supervising visit telling the registered nurse that the patient already fell that morning during the bath visit.

HOME HEALTH CARE AND/OR HOSPICE TEAM CONFERENCES

There may be times when you are requested to meet at the office or in the home of a patient for a formal team conference. Team conferences are meetings held to discuss the patient's situation, progress, or lack of progress. Aides are involved whenever possible because as front line caregivers, their opinions and observations are important and a necessary part of the decision making process about the future care of the patient. Hospice has what are called "IDT" meetings or interdisciplinary team meetings. For more information readers are referred to the "Hospice Care" guidelines.

As an example, the aide may have observed that the patient needs less personal care assistance than what was needed at the beginning of the case. This information will provide the team with direct knowledge that the patient has improved and may be ready to be discharged from home care. The aide's opinions and input do make a difference, as they may identify the need for and suggest: physical or occupational therapy, medical social services to evaluate family dynamics and finances, or speech-language pathology. Other services may also be appropriate to improve patient independence or functioning. The aide usually spends the most time with patients and may be in the best position to make recommendations for additional patient care assistance.

At patient care conferences, patient information is shared and the patient's status is updated and documented. The aide may be asked to assist with the documentation or provide an update in the patient's status. The interchange of communication is the purpose of these conferences. Other services identified as being needed, such as nutritional, volunteer, or chaplain services, or a date for projected discharge, may be discussed. This is also the time that patient complications, problems, or other needs are identified. All of these patient care communications, whether in person, at a team meeting, or on the phone, contribute to meeting the needs identified on the patient's individualized care plan. Some organizations also communicate by way of a communication sheet left in the home.

The nurses and therapists depend upon the aide to immediately communicate to them any change in patient's status. Emergency communication numbers, either in the patient's home or on the aide assignment sheet, should include agency office numbers, after hours and on-call phone numbers, and any appropriate beeper or voice mail numbers. In the home, emergency phone numbers should also include family work and home numbers, as well as local emergency medical assistance phone numbers. It is important to emphasize to the patient and family which important numbers should be posted. This would include the organization's number, on-call number, 911 or other local number to access emergency services, and the physician's phone number.

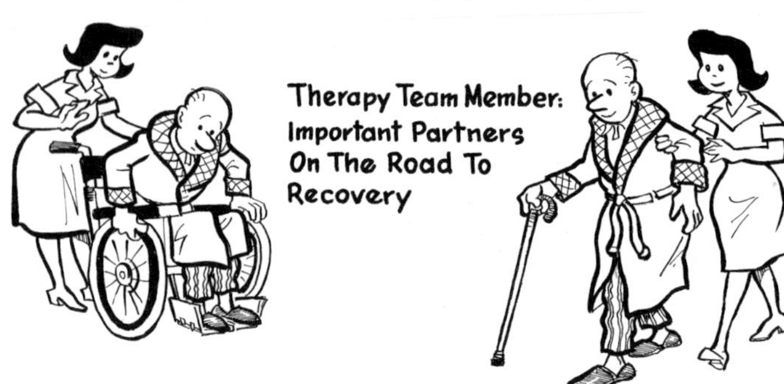

COMMUNICATIONS WITH PATIENTS AND THEIR FAMILIES

The relationship that has been established between the aide and the patient and family is so personal, that patients may get upset when there is a schedule change, regardless of the reason. Some patients may make negative comments about another aide, other agency staff, and family members. It is important to listen to patients, but do not support or discuss negative or rude comments made by the patient about your co-workers or others. Many times patterns of negative communication have become habit and occurred before the home care team became involved. The family may be upset due to the stress of the illness. Or, the family may not be coping with the long-term issues associated with the patient's care. Sometimes patients get accustomed to the patterns of one aide, and may find it difficult to adjust to new people. Negative remarks or behaviors may need to be reported to your supervisor, as noted in organization protocols. Support the supervisor during the investigation, but maintain strict confidentiality.

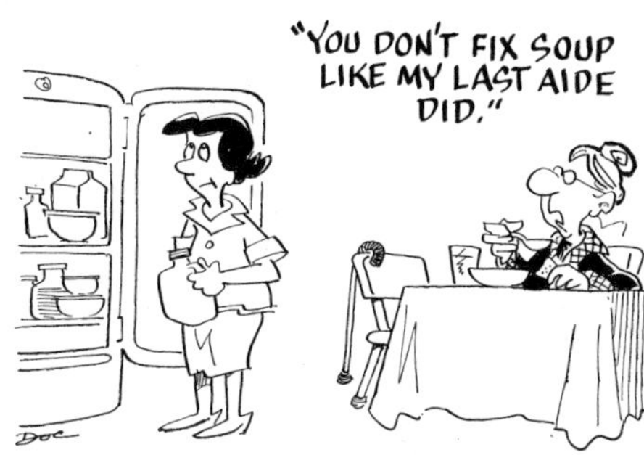

WORKING WITH OTHER PROGRAMS TO MEET PATIENT NEEDS

A patient also may receive services from other agencies or organizations. At times, your supervisor may not be aware of new developments or referrals made outside of the organization's system. Examples of these services could be Meals on Wheels, volunteer support programs, or other local community services. An example of this situation would be the patient who is placed on hold status, pending a hospital readmission, and is discharged home over the weekend to the services of another home care program. The aide from the first organization makes a scheduled visit and finds that a nurse from another organization is already providing patient services. It is the responsibility of the aide to notify the supervisor so that this duplication of services can be addressed and resolved.

When communicating about the patient with your supervisor or the patient care manager, be sure to

"WE'RE PLAYING 'MEALS ON WHEELS'."

discuss all other services involved in the patient's plan of care, to make your manager aware of all organizations providing services. This will assist with the coordination of services while helping to avoid confusion for your patient about the different organizations. Any questions that the other program's staff asks about those services or programs the patient should be referred to your supervisor.

SUMMARY

In summary, the team effort in home and hospice care is key to meeting patient needs. Care coordination is an important part of communication with all home care team members. The team concept includes communications with patients, their caregivers, and other disciplines and team members involved in the patient's care. The active participation of the aide in patient care communications is vital to help the team provide appropriate and high quality care. The aides do this effectively by addressing the personal care, the day-to-day needs of patients and their caregivers.

REVIEW EXERCISES

1) Define the home health care team. (See page 38).
2) Define the hospice team. (See page 38-39)
3) Explain one reason for home care or hospice team conference. (See page 38-39).
4) State the reason for the home health aide care plan or assignment sheet. (See page 40).
5) List the five services involved in Mr. Able's care. Briefly explain why they are involved.
(See page 41, 42, 43).
6) Describe why communication and coordination among/between team members is so important to patient care and safety in both home health care and hospice (See page 43-44).

CHAPTER FIVE

HOME HEALTH CARE DOCUMENTATION REQUIREMENTS

Documentation in home health care and in hospice is very important for many reasons. The documentation about patients is kept in the organization's clinical or medical records. The clinical information or documentation about the patient's progress is confidential information that provides communication to the doctor, the insurance company, case managers, your supervisor, and other team members about the patient's care. For all of these reasons, it is important that the care (including the aide's care) matches the care ordered.

WHY IS DOCUMENTATION SO IMPORTANT?

Important Reasons For A Clinical Record Include:

1) It is the only written source for communication and reference for members of the home health care team.
2) It supports payment for insurance coverage or denial for provided patient care services.
3) It is the source for review and evaluation of the care provided.
4) It is a legal record.
5) It is important to maintaining organization certification or accreditation.

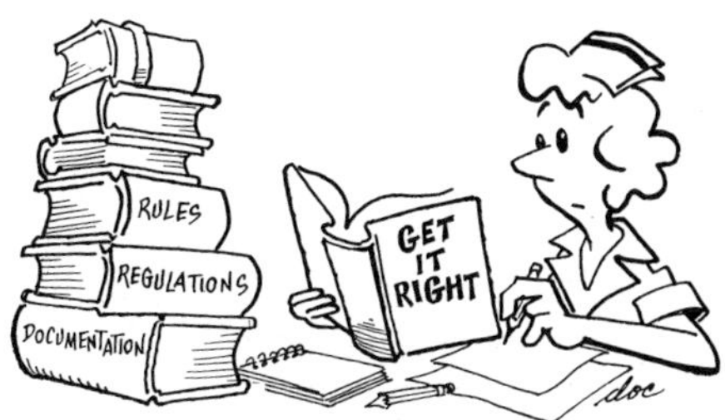

RULES ABOUT
DOCUMENTATION: THE BASICS

Certain rules need to be followed when completing documentation for the clinical record. Aide documentation reports what was done and occurred during the visit. Effective documentation practice includes the following:

- List the patient's name and your number, if applicable, according to your organization's protocol.
- Report on each assigned task or duty (as noted on the aide assignment form) for each visit or shift.
- Complete patient note for every shift or visit.
- Finish the documentation as soon as the work is completed (e.g., as soon as the work is completed, write it on the visit/shift record prior to leaving the patient's home.)
- Record any patient refusal to have a task performed, along with the reason, if given, on the visit note and make sure to notify your supervisor.
- Speak with the supervisor, if in doubt about any documentation issues.
- Your patient may be asked to sign or initial the visit documentation or other agency form.

DOCUMENTATION TIPS

- Print neatly or write legibly.
- Use black or blue ink, not pencil (your organization may specify a preferred color of ink).
- For every note, identify the patient's name, the time of arrival, and departure and date.
- Sign each note and include your title after your name (e.g., aide, CHHA, CNA).
- Be factual, accurate, and specific.
- Chart only the care you provided.
- Avoid relying on memory.
- Do not make assumptions, draw conclusions, or asign blame.
- Ask your supervisor for any documentation policies and procedures at your organization.
- Correct mistakes as per organization policy.
- Notes should show that the aide follows the assignment
- If your organization uses an automatic call-in system for attendance and documentation, you will be instructed on its use. Ask your supervisor if you don't know how to document something.

Other Tips:

____

____

____

THE SUPERVISOR'S REVIEW
OF YOUR DOCUMENTATION

Patient notes may be reviewed by the supervisor. Narrative and checklist notes show the actual care provided to patients. This review is a common part of an important process called "quality improvement" (QI) or performance improvement (PI). These are ongoing processes that continually strive to improve patient care and organizational operations. It may include supervisory visits of care in the home, documentation reviews, patient satisfaction surveys, and physician comments.

ABOUT DOCUMENTATION,
ACCREDITATION, AND QUALITY

You may be caring for a patient when a surveyor or site visitor comes with the nurse to meet with your patient. These visitors can be from accreditation organizations, such as the Joint Commission on Accreditation of Healthcare Organizations (JCAHO), the Community Health Accreditation Program (CHAP), The Accreditation Commission for Healthcare (ACHC). Accreditation organizations define national standards for care and organizational quality improvement initiatives. The accreditations surveyors visit to validate that specific standards are met by accredited organizations. Surveyors or site visitors could be from the state or federal agencies, or from your own organization's QI team.

Accreditation requires QI or PI and home visits; it is one of the ways of assessing the quality of care patients receive from an organization. The home health aide documentation assists in demonstrating the provision of safe and effective personal care to patients. This is an important part of any accreditation or regulatory review of the organization's operations related to patient care.

WHAT TO DOCUMENT: SUPPORTING PROFESSIONALISM

It is important that your documentation match the information on the aide assignment sheet or care plan and instructions by the nurse. To any record reviewer, the documentation should paint a clear picture of the patient's condition and the needs that require your special care. The information should be factual and objective because the clinical documentation is the paper trail of the care provided and the patient's response to that care.

Again, in your documentation, it is important not to be judgmental about your patient's lifestyle choices or cultural background. For example: "I kept telling Mrs. Smith not to smoke and now she's coming out of the hospital again with pneumonia." A better documentation would be "Mrs. Smith reports that she just came home from the hospital with pneumonia. Aide called office at 2:00 p.m. and informed the supervisor that when she arrived, the patient was smoking in the home without supervision."

Your home care or hospice organization may have examples of documentation for you to review to improve your documentation. Your agency may also have examples of effective notes or correctly completed checklists.

DOCUMENTATION EXAMPLES

Here are some examples of documentation. Notice the difference between the first two and last two notes.

The first two notes provide specific information related to the patient's mobility and medication compliance. Note that when a change in the patient's skin was observed, it was reported to the nurse right away with the time and the nurse to whom the problem was reported.

The second two notes demonstrate inappropriate documentation. Health care workers should not express an opinion on a paper that is part of the patient's clinical record. The aide should not administer medications (ear drops) and always should follow the organization's policy regarding medications.

2 EXAMPLES OF WRITING RIGHT

7/15 8:30 AM Morning care performed. Ambulated in corridor with walker. BM today. Took meds in morning slot. Red area on coccyx reported to nurse Sarah Smith. **Sally Murphy, HHA**

7/15 11:00 AM Morning care done including shampoo. ROM excercises done. Absorbent underpad changed 2x. Drank coffee and juice with help. No BM today. **Martin Jones, HHA**

2 EXAMPLES OF WHAT NOT TO WRITE

7/15 9:00 AM Assisted with shower. Nurse should have ordered shower chair as pt. was very shaky. This lady should be in a nursing home.
Cindy Smith, HHA

7/15 Assisted with shave, foot soak. C/O earache + put drops in ears. **Dana Byer, HHA**

SUMMARY

It is important to remember that documentation is the paper trail of the care provided and the patient's response to that care. Effective clinical documentation paints a picture of the patient and the care provided. When writing clinical documentation keep in mind that effective documentation addresses two important standards:

1) It demonstrates the care that was provided to the patient.
2) It is required by Medicare, accreditation, and other regulatory bodies.

REVIEW EXERCISES

1) List three reasons why the clinical record is important. (See page 50).
2) Describe three ways to document effectively. (See page 51).
3) Where is the documentation kept? (See page 50).
4) Identify two basic rules about documentation. (See page 51).
5) Name four documentation tips. (See page 52).

CHAPTER SIX

SUPERVISION IN HOME CARE (OR HOW TO BE VALUED BY MANAGEMENT)

Supervision of home health or hospice aides is a required or mandated standard of practice in home or hospice care. It is a quality measure for your patients and their families. Some programs supervise aides every two weeks, a homemaker once a month, and others more or less often. This schedule is based on the patient's needs, contractual arrangements, and regulations. Your supervisor may visit while you are with the patient or meet with the patient and family when the aide is not there. The coordination of scheduling visit times with both the nurse and the aide can be difficult and tests the skills of both the scheduling coordinator and the nurse supervisors. At some time during the course of working with the patient, you will probably be making joint visits with the patient's nurse, therapist, or supervising nurse. All team members are supervised by either their supervisor or another team member to monitor quality.

ABOUT JOINT HOME VISITS

The nurse or therapist will be reviewing the patient's care plan to determine if there is a need to delete or add particular tasks or duties, based on the patient's individual needs and problems. These needs are identified during the nurse's or therapist's assessment/reassessment and/or during patient and caregiver interviews. In addition, the nurse supervisor or therapist may observe the aide in the actual provision of personal care or while assisting patients with their ADLs. The nurse supervisor or therapist may provide teaching and training to the aide during the joint home visits. These various supervisory responsibilities are required and help to assure the quality of care your home care or hospice organization provides.

OTHER SUPERVISORY COMMUNICATIONS

Phone call supervision may also occur on a regular or random basis when the supervisor calls the patient or family to check on the patient's status and asks for feedback about the care provided. Patients are consumers of care and are customers of the home care organization. The aide should do all that is reasonable to assure that patient needs are met, as well as keep patients happy with our services. We must do our part, our best, to try and meet this important goal of patient satisfaction. In fact, most home care and hospice organizations send out a questionnaire or a "survey" form to patients to assess patient satisfaction in order to identify ways to improve services and care. Through these methods of communication, we can see the importance of home visits and joint visits with nurses and other supervisors to try to provide the most effective service and care possible.

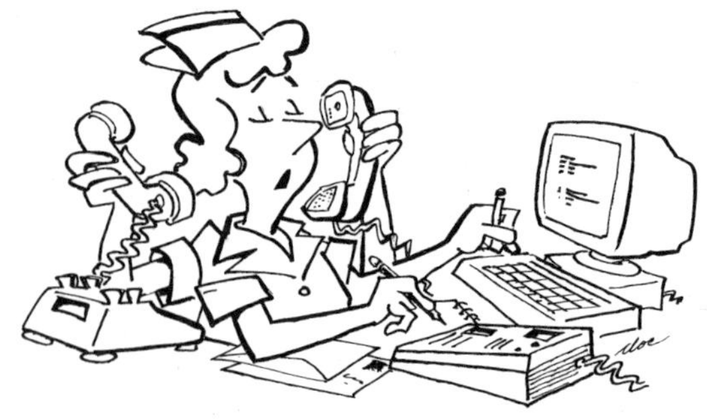

SCHEDULING CONSIDERATIONS

Many times the supervisor or scheduling coordinator (who may be a nurse) will match patients and aides based on various criteria, i.e., skill matching, which is an important part of supervision. Scheduling is a very important part of supervision from the manager's perspective. It is important that the aide adhere to this schedule to effectively provide patient care. It is for this reason that tardiness should be avoided. Additionally, effective scheduling includes informing the patient of how often, and what time, various home care team members will be making a visit. Schedule changes should be communicated by a representative of the organization based on the organization's policies and procedures related to schedule changes. Patient schedule changes can only occur if your supervisor approves it. In general, all communications should go through your organization and your supervisor. To avoid any confusion, misunderstandings and problems, do not give your home or beeper number to your patients. Be aware that with the addition of caller identification (or "ID"), patients/family members would now (after calling) have your personal phone number.

**The following information is considered
when making the schedule:**

- Skill level required
- Patient needs
- Aide availability
- Punctuality
- Travel
- Time availability
- Geographical location
- Weather conditions
- Patient schedule changes
- Sick callouts

- Patient refusal of entry or care
- The patient's diagnosis and the aide's expertise or experience
- Other considerations

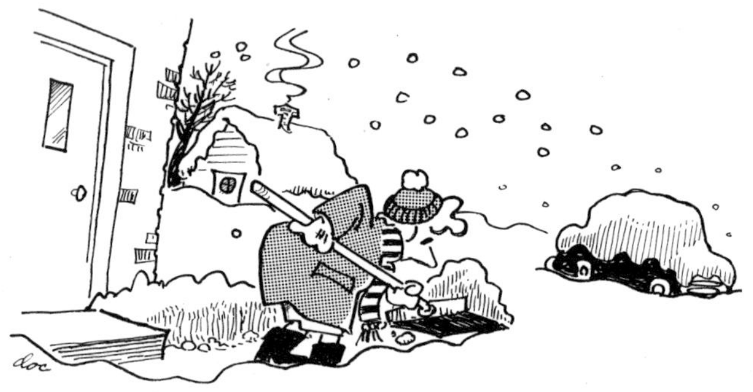

SCHEDULING EXAMPLE
BASED ON PATIENT NEED

Most patients want to have personal care needs completed in the early morning. However, scheduling is based upon the individual needs of all the patients in relation to the ability of the organization to meet requests for services. An example of scheduling based on priority is the paraplegic patient who needs personal care early in the morning in order to get to work on time (This is a patient where "homebound" is not a requirement.). This is an example of a patient whose needs make it imperative that the aide make a visit early in the morning. In contrast, a bed bound patient's care plan may not require the provision of personal care at any specific time during the day. Follow your organization's policies to inform your patient of the appropriate time of your visit.

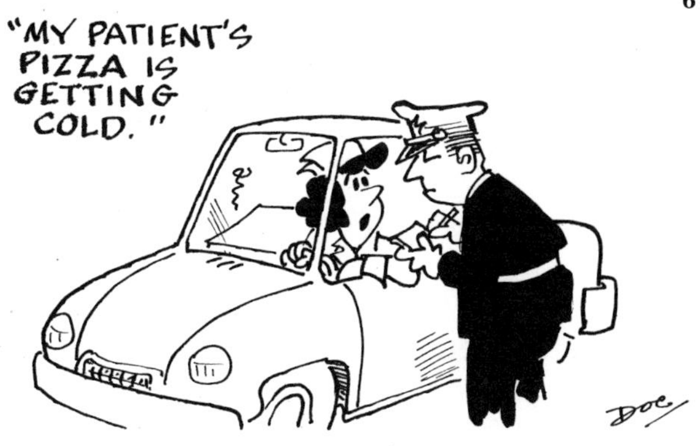

CHANGES IN SCHEDULING

Changes in times, duties, or other previously agreed upon arrangements cannot occur without permission from your supervisor. There must be communication with the office for any changes related to patient care visits, times, and responsibilities, other than those previously scheduled. Team members such as the OT, PT, SLP, MSS, dietitians, and others usually plan their visits around the aide's schedule. Because of this, it is imperative that the schedule not be changed without communicating those changes to affected team members. If you complete your assignment early, or the patient wants you to leave, ask to use the phone to call your supervisor about the change. Aides may be asked to "fill in" for other aides from time to time. In this instance, your patients should always be notified of any changes.

WORKING TOWARD DISCHARGE

The aide supervisor informs the aide of the anticipated patient discharge date from the organization. Saying goodbye to your patients can be very difficult. Throughout the time care is provided, the nurses and other team members should prepare the patient for eventual discharge from services. All team members need to consider and plan for how the patient will manage after services are withdrawn. Discharge should not be a surprise to patients and their family members or to the home health aide. It is usually a planned event and is dependent on effective communications by all involved. For example, once the patient is assessed by the nurse, the nurse or therapist may predict a timeline and estimated discharge date on the initial visit, when possible. Often, the number of visits decreases as the discharge date approaches and the patient's needs diminish. This discharge information is important, as it assists you in encouraging and allowing patients to do more for themselves. Usually, it is also the role of the nurse or the therapist to inform or communicate this information to the patient. Discharge from home care services should never be a surprise to patients, their families, or caregivers. Effective discharge planning and care coordination prevent this unfortunate occurrence.

SAYING GOODBYE TO YOUR PATIENTS

Saying goodbye to your patients can be difficult and sometimes personally painful. It is important that these feelings are discussed with your supervisor, particularly in difficult or long-term cases. In this way you may be able to avoid any possible problems that may arise from your close or long-term relationship. In reality, home care team members don't always get to say goodbye to their patients, family, or friends. This may happen when a patient suddenly has to be hospitalized and does not return home, or if the patient dies between care visits. In these instances, you may want to talk to your supervisor about your feelings of loss, sadness or other uncomfortable emotions.

SUMMARY

Your positive working relationship with your supervisor is important for effective communication in home care. Your relationship with your supervisor and the home care organization impact patient care through the daily schedule, assigned tasks, and patient care changes, all of which must be communicated to be effective.

In conclusion, the aide must communicate changes in visit times, duties, or other previously agreed upon arrangements, as these require permission from your supervisor. Your use of positive and effective interpersonal communication skills will assist in these changes while contributing to safe patient care.

REVIEW EXERCISES

1) What is a joint visit? (See page 57).
2) List four scheduling considerations. Describe the challenges they present for covering the organization's caseload. (See page 59-60).
3) When should the projected discharge date be determined? (See page 62).
4) What are the feelings that may arise when discharging a patient with whom you've developed a close or long-term relationship? (See page 62).
5) Your patient's family complains to you that "The other aide just sits around and doesn't make my meal like you do." What should the aide do?
(A reply and an action.)

CHAPTER SEVEN

SAFETY IN HOME HEALTH CARE

PERSONAL SAFETY: AN OVERVIEW

Personal safety is important to us all, but especially to those who enter geographical areas with which they may not be familiar and at unusual hours. Your organization wants to assure your safety during visits. Be aware of any particular safety measures or protocols that should be explained during your orientation. Personal safety starts with you. Whenever you are going anywhere for the first time, mentally drive or walk yourself to the home. Get specific directions, ask about parking, and whether you need to call first. Lock the car doors, especially the driver's side door and keep any valuables out of sight or, preferably, at home.

As you are driving, always be aware of your surroundings. Wear your seat belt and follow state laws regarding seat belts. Their use is mandatory in many states and may also be part of your organization's safety policies. Ask your supervisor about this requirement. When you are nearing the home, look for the landmarks described, or address numbers on houses. Once at the home, lock your car, making sure no items noting patient's names are visible. Be cautious when boarding an elevator. If other passengers appear suspicious, get off and wait for another elevator or take other actions, based on your judgment of the situation. Before getting into your car, check the backseat and floorboard areas. Your supplies, purse, and bag should be kept out of sight in the car.

If you are uncomfortable or feel unsafe in a home or particular environment, discuss this with your supervisor, so that precautions can be taken to enhance your safety. Speak with your supervisor about your organization's policies and procedures related to safety in your community.

CAR SAFETY: TAKING CARE OF YOUR CAR

Car safety begins with familiarizing yourself with the strengths and weaknesses of your car. Making sure you have enough gas is only the first step. Other car safety hints include:

- Carry one gallon of water, a blanket, a first aid kit, and a flashlight.
- Lock all doors immediately upon entering or leaving the car.
- Carry sand, kitty litter, or rug mats to assist you out of snow and ice.
- Use your sign identifying you as a home health care worker, per program policies.
- Consider obtaining a gasoline credit card instead of carrying cash.
- Take care of your car: winterize it and maintain it.
- Carry a small fire extinguisher.
- Check oil and fluid levels (like windshield washer fluid) regularly.
- Others, recommended by your supervisor, organization, or employer.

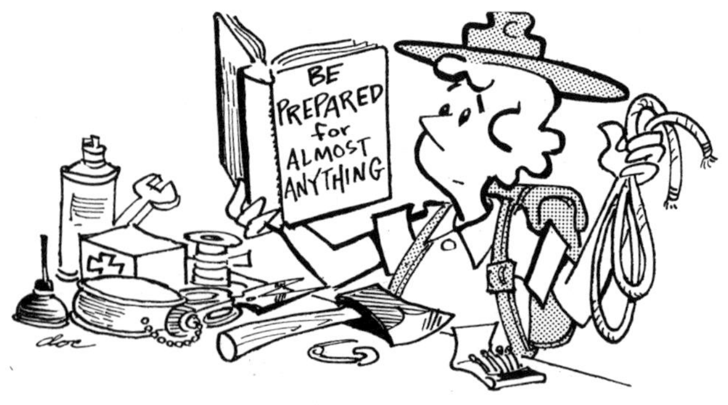

PERSONAL SAFETY CONSIDERATIONS

- Park in well lit areas, as close to your destination as possible.
- Make sure your spare tire is inflated and your tires are in good condition.
- When approaching your car, have your keys out, ready to unlock your car.
- Consider joining an automotive association such as AAA for assistance in emergencies with towing, gasoline, and dead batteries.
- Try to maintain at least half a tank of gas. Do not make visits running on empty.
- Place your equipment bag where it is not visible.
- Have detailed and correct directions to the patient's home.
- Keep maps out of sight. Try to avoid looking as though you are unfamiliar with the area.
- When making evening visits, let your family know when they should expect you to return.
- If you have one, keep your mobile/cell phone ready for use.
- Monitor your pager.
- Avoid carrying a purse or valuables and carry only the essentials.
- Wear ID badge at all times.
- Any falls/injuries during work time should be reported ASAP to your supervisor.
- Other recommendations by your supervisor, organization, or employer.

MAP READING

Another necessary skill for home health care workers is effective map reading. Whether you own your own map book or have copies of the pages you need, your ability to navigate about many towns will be tested. You will find yourself noting landmarks, schools, playgrounds, shopping areas, etc. that help you to direct or be directed to patient's homes. Your personal safety depends on your ability to get easily from one patient to the next. Ask your supervisor about your organization's geographic or "catchment" area for any information you may need to more effectively and safely get from home to home. For example, on certain days, the street cleaners may come through and no parking is allowed, or streets with multiple lanes change in direction to accommodate rush hour traffic. If you use the bus system or other public transportation, be aware of schedules and changes due to weather and other problems that affect your visit schedule.

SAFE AND EFFECTIVE BODY MECHANICS: USE OF A TRANSFER BELT

When you provide physical assistance to patients, it's a good idea to use a transfer belt when:

- Transferring from bed to chair and back
- Ambulating patients about the home
- Providing transfer assistance in and out of the shower/tub
- Assisting family to transfer in/out of vehicle
- Climbing stairs
- Other activities that require lifting and may cause back strain

- Keep your back straight. Bend at the knees and lift with your legs. Do not bend forward at the hips.

The transfer belt may be provided by your organization with instructions for its use. Report any loss or breakage of the transfer belt, as it is a very important piece of equipment. The use of the transfer belt and safe body mechanics help to keep your back strong. Remember to always lift following agency policy. Also, always adjust the bed height to turn and position as well as to change the linens.

SUMMARY

Safety in home health care and hospice is important to all team members. Your safety is very important to your organization. Personal safety, car safety, and safe moving and lifting begin with you. Ask your supervisor for more specific policies and procedures related to safety issues.

REVIEW EXERCISES

1) List three safety considerations to keep in mind when you are going somewhere for the first time. (See page 65).
2) Identify four car safety tips. (See page 66).
3) Name three instances when a transfer belt should be used. (See page 68).
4) Explain why map reading is a necessary skill for home health or hospice aides (See page 68).
5) List three topics that are "safety related" that were addressed by your employer/organization in an inservice or during orientation.

CHAPTER EIGHT

INFECTION CONTROL IN
HOME HEALTH CARE

There has been much media coverage related to infection control and health care. Topics such as the avian or bird flu and resistant organisms or "bugs" are frequently in the newspaper or reported in the news. You have an important role to play in stopping the transmission of infection.

Infections are diseases that are caused by bacteria or viruses and are invisible to the human eye. Infections spread when the organisms (bacteria and viruses) are "carried" from one site (or person) to another. **For example, organisms can get on our hands and be passed either to ourselves or to another person who we touch with our hands. This makes hand washing the most important way to prevent spreading infection.** The organisms in our environment can be spread in different ways and do not always make us sick, nevertheless we must always be alert to protect ourselves and our patients. The term "standard precautions" describes the methods we use to protect ourselves and our patients from these invisible germs and organisms.

STANDARD PRECAUTIONS

Many infections are spread before it is known that they are present, or before people show symptoms that they are even sick. For that reason all health care workers must use standard precautions to protect themselves and their patients, and decrease the spread of infections. *Standard precautions are guidelines to be used when taking care of any patient.* These precautions are the best way to protect ourselves and our patients from the spread of infections. ***Standard precautions*** include:

- Effective hand washing – ***before*** and ***after*** care of each patient, and after using the bathroom anywhere. Wearing gloves does not negate the need for frequent hand washing. Wash your hands after removing gloves.
- Use of gloves – gloves should be used with any hands-on patient contact, i.e., bathing, use of bed pans, commodes, drainage bags, handling of feces, urine, vomitus, blood, and equipment.
- Use of other personal protective equipment (PPE) as required by the patient's unique condition – goggles, masks, face coverings, aprons, foot coverings, gowns.
- Use of cleaning liquids – alcohol, bleach, peroxide, white vinegar. Make sure to follow proper ratios, like 1:10 for bleach to water. Always be careful using patient's bleach in the patient's household.
- Continuing education such as in-service education on a regular basis to teach all staff when and how to utilize all equipment available to protect themselves and their patients.

Standard precautions are effective and important tools to use to prevent and control the spread of any organism or infection. When properly used, there should be no fear of spreading organisms from patient to patient, or from staff member to other staff or family. This also includes knowing when you are sick and getting advice as to whether or not you should go to work. For instance, you may have a cold and not really be sick enough to need to stay home. However, you may need to use a mask when caring for your patients to prevent your (already sick) patients from catching your cold. It is important to note that colds are viruses and may spread by droplet through coughing, touching your face, sneezing, handling tissues, etc. Always wash your hands more frequently with the onset of a cold or other symptoms. This is especially true during the annual flu season!

Organizations should supply soap and paper towels or waterless hand products or sanitizers to their staff for use in the event the patient's home has none. Aides must be responsible to keep supplies on hand and should ask their organization what the policies are related to hand washing supplies. Do not use soiled, used towels or bar soap in a patient's home. Any equipment, gloves, masks, gowns, or paper towels, must be disposed of according to your organization's policy. A wastebasket with a disposable paper or plastic bag is usually appropriate.

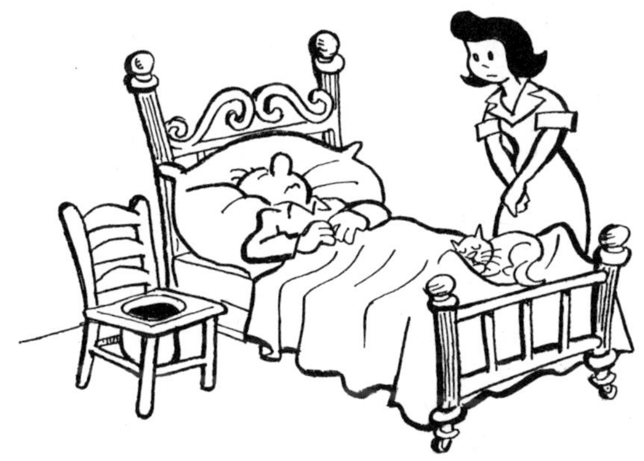

ABOUT OSHA

The Occupational Safety and Health Administration (OSHA) is the department of the United States government that is responsible for defining occupational safety and enforcing safety laws for all workers. Since the health care industry can involve possible exposure to some infections, we must always be alert to possible sources and symptoms of infection.

Standard precautions are a method or an approach to

infection control including prevention and protection guidelines outlined by OSHA. The home care organization should always have proper personal protective equipment available to staff. This equipment includes disposable gloves, masks, aprons or other coverings, and mouth pieces for CPR and other equipment as necessary. The nurse will communicate any specific symptoms or precautions to be alert to with each patient. The nurse should also identify any special protective equipment which will be necessary for care. Always be sure to wash your hands before you start your work at each home and just as you are leaving. Additional hand washing should occur before and after food preparation, bathing, or any personal care tasks. When in doubt, wash your hands. Remember that warm water, soap, scrubbing, rinsing, and wiping dry with a clean cloth or towels are some of the most effective deterrents to (ways to control) the transmission of germs.

Organisms can be spread several ways:

1) **Airborne** – passed from one place or person to another through the air, such as through sneezing or coughing. Examples of airborne diseases are measles and tuberculosis.

2) **Sexual** – passed during sexual contact like "wet" kissing (kissing with an exchange of body fluids), sexual intercourse, or other sexual behaviors. Examples include herpes, hepatitis B, HIV, syphilis, and chlamydia.

3) **Oral** – passed from one person to another by sharing of food or drinks. This method can pass infection from one person to an other.

4) **Handling** – the most frequent way to spread infection when proper hand washing is not used. An example of an infection passed by improper handling is E. Coli (an organism present in fecal matter or feces).

5) **Sharing** – using razors, drinks, ointments, toothbrushes, etc.

CLEANING PATIENT SUPPLIES

Before using any cleaning protocols or procedures, check with your supervisor about your agency's specific policies and procedures for guidance and direction. In addition, other supplies, such as biohazardous bags, may be required based on the soiled or spilled material and your organization's policies and procedures. When in doubt, always check with your supervisor.

For infection control and safety reasons, it is important that the patient area and supplies be kept clean. When you first meet the patient, ask the nurse about the care and cleaning of any equipment in the home. Equipment you might be asked to keep clean include:

- Oxygen humidifier bottle – Clean with soap and water, then allow to dry before re-using.
- Urine collection bags - Clean with white vinegar solution (one part white vinegar to three parts water, i.e., one cup white vinegar to three cups water), rinse with plain water, air-dry until next use.
- Plastic equipment – Bedpans, urinals, emesis basins, commodes. These should be cleaned with soap and water, using a brush as needed (the same brush should not be used for any other purpose). Allow to air dry.
- Metal equipment – Walkers, canes, wheelchairs may need to be wiped down occasionally with soap and water, especially if they have been soiled by a body fluid.
- Soiled paper products and dressing supplies – These should be placed in a paper bag or plastic bag (per your agency's policy), tied closed and then in a plastic bag, and tied closed. This is called double bagging. Dispose of material in a trash can. Ask your supervisor for your organization's policy for additional information about disposing of soiled products or dressings.
- Sharp items – These should be contained in a hard

plastic container, preferably a container designed for needle/lancet disposal. Whenever possible, have the patient dispose of the sharp item by handing the container to the patient for disposal, rather than taking the sharp item from the patient and disposing of it yourself. **Never recap needles.** Ask to review your organization's policies and procedures relating to infection control, sharps disposal, and other items. This includes lancets, used to prick fingers for blood sugar readings.

- Soiled linen – Soiled linen should be handled wearing gloves and holding them at arm's length away from your own clothing or uniform. Wear an apron, when possible. Place soiled linen directly in a laundry bag or the washing machine.

- Blood spills – Wear gloves when cleaning blood spills, using bleach solution (one part bleach to ten parts water). Again, ask your supervisor for specific directions that may be unique to your patient or your program. Bleach packets may be supplied for staff to carry.

GENERAL HYGIENE TIPS

Other Items To Remember:

- Whenever possible, and weather permitting, open windows to allow fresh air into the patient's home. When opening windows, consider safety of the neighborhood. Remember to close windows before leaving the home since the patient/family may have difficulty closing them and/or forget about the open windows.

- Never share personal articles between people. This includes combs, razors, toothbrushes, towels, etc.

- Some patients should not eat raw foods (salad, raw eggs) or drink tap water in certain parts of the country. Check with the nurse about any dietary or other restrictions.

- Always wash your hands thoroughly after handling pets. Some patients should not change litter boxes, bird cages, or aquariums because of organisms that are carried by such animals in their feces can cause diseases in humans. Again, check with the nurse about your patient's specific care plan and needs.
- Keep your fingernails short and clean, to safely and comfortably provide personal and other care. (And do not wear/use acrylic nails for work.)
- Keep cuts or any broken skin areas covered and protected and wear latex gloves when providing any personal care.
- Attend organizational or employer sponsored in-services to learn more about: AIDS care, Herpes Zoster (shingles), infection control and standard precautions, tuberculosis, symptoms of infections like pneumonia, urinary tract infections, wound infections, etc. This important information will also assist you in your personal, professional, and family life.

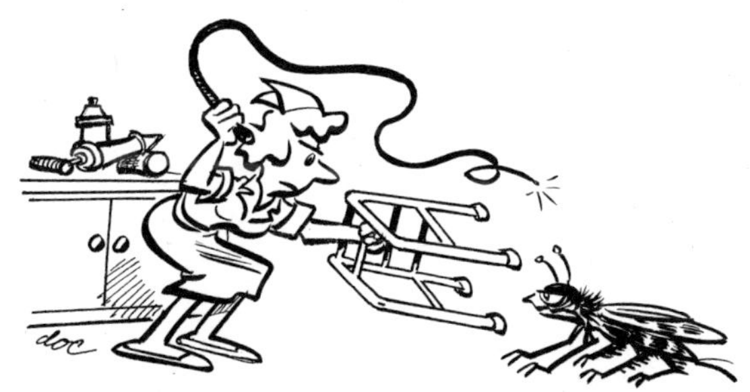

OTHER HOME HEALTH CARE INFECTION CONTROL CONSIDERATIONS

- Report any insects and rodents in the patient's home to the nurse and/or supervisor.
- Store sterile solutions like saline in the refrigerator or per organizational policies.

- Report any animal or human bites immediately.
- Report any exposure to bodily fluids, secretions, or needle sticks to your supervisor immediately.
- Report to the nurse or supervisor when supplies are low or equipment is not working properly, or when cleaning solutions are not available.
- Do not apply lipbalm or lipstick in a patient's home or when hands need washing.
- Keep your patient care bag and any equipment clean and organized (see bag technique).
- Place any specimens you are asked to obtain in a clear plastic bag, preferably in a ziplock type or one that has been provided by your organization, and transport or carry upright in a puncture resistant container approved by your supervisor.
- Clean or assist patients to clean their hands after bathroom use, and before eating.
- If an object is "wet", don't touch it without wearing gloves.
- Keep pets out of the patient care area when caring for the patient (when possible).
- Discard protective equipment after one use.
- Store ointments used for the patient away from those used by other family members.
- Take care of yourself by eating properly, exercising, getting enough sleep, practicing effective hygiene and infection control and allowing for time away from the job.
- Wash your hands! Wash your hands! Wash your hands!

EFFECTIVE HAND WASHING: A REVIEW

Hand washing is something that we do so frequently that we may tend to forget its importance. **Hand washing is probably the most important step in stopping the transmission of infection. When in doubt, wash your**

hands. The steps to proper hand washing include:
- Use liquid soap, rather than a bar of soap, whenever possible.
- Use paper towels to dry your hands or a clean cloth towel when paper is not available.
- Remove rings.
- Vigorously lather hands with soap and warm water, wash between fingers, under nails, and the wrist area. (Rinsing with water alone is not enough!)
- Turn off the faucet(s) with a paper towel after hand washing.
- Properly dispose of paper towels.

Effective hand washing is the responsibility of all home care personnel. Some organizations supply individual containers of soap and packages of paper towels. These should be stored in your equipment bag. At the beginning of each visit, remove the soap and towels from your bag for use during the visit. Before you leave, wash your hands, using the above procedure, and replace the soap and towels in your bag. Repeat this procedure at all homes you visit. Waterless soap products may be used when soap and water are not available. Follow the manufacturer's directions.

INFECTION CONTROL AND YOUR HOME CARE BAG

HHAs may use a zippered bag to contain equipment for patient care use. It is the responsibility of each HHA to keep this equipment clean and properly stored. Restock items as needed.

- Never place contaminated or dirty or used articles in your bag.
- There may be distinct "clean" and "dirty" sections in your bag.

- Store equipment for convenience. Gloves, soap, and water should be near the top.
- Always close the bag when not in use.
- Keep the bag where you can see it during the visit, if possible - - and not on the floor!
- Place the bag on top of a newspaper or paper towel when in the home.
- Be aware that pets may try to get inside or lie on top of your bag. Keep it closed.
- When in a home that has insects or rodents, do not bring your bag into the home. Only bring in those items (such as soap and towels) that will be needed for that particular patient's care.
- Follow your organization's policies and procedures regarding infection control of stethoscopes, blood pressure cuffs, and other patient supply items.

SUMMARY

Infections are caused by germs, bacteria and viruses and are invisible to the human eye. Infections are "carried" from one site, object, or person to another. This makes hand washing the most important way to prevent the spread of infection. The term "standard precautions" describes the methods used to protect ourselves and our patients from these invisible germs, viruses, and organisms. Your organization's infection control policies define specific procedures and supplies that may be used for infection control. The home health or hospice aide is in an important position to help stop the spread of infection.

REVIEW EXERCISES

1) What is the most important way to prevent the spread of infection? (See page 78).
2) Define "standard precautions" and identify for which patients they are used. (See page 71).
3) Describe the role of OSHA regarding health care workers and their safety. (See page 73-74).
4) Name four general hygiene tips. (See page 76-77).
5) Describe the steps in effective handwashing (See page 78-79).
6) Demonstrate effective hand washing/hand hygiene per organizational policy.

CHAPTER NINE

ADMINISTRATIVE RESPONSIBILITIES

YOUR ROLE IN UPDATING YOUR HUMAN RESOURCE OR PERSONNEL FILE

After completing the aide certification course, you probably thought that your education was complete. However, all health care workers must regularly review old (or known) information or learn new skills to maintain proficiency and competency. This includes reading information, listening to audiotapes, reviewing videotapes, going online, or attending in-service education programs. Some agencies may provide these in-service programs on the computer. By keeping up-to-date on current information or learning new skills, we continue to ensure that we will do the best possible job of taking care of our patients. Medicare requires that home health aides receive at least 12 hours of in-service training during each 12 month period. Some of this in-service training may occur while you are furnishing care to the patient. Ask your supervisor or employer about your specific education requirements. The state you practice in may have additional requirements.

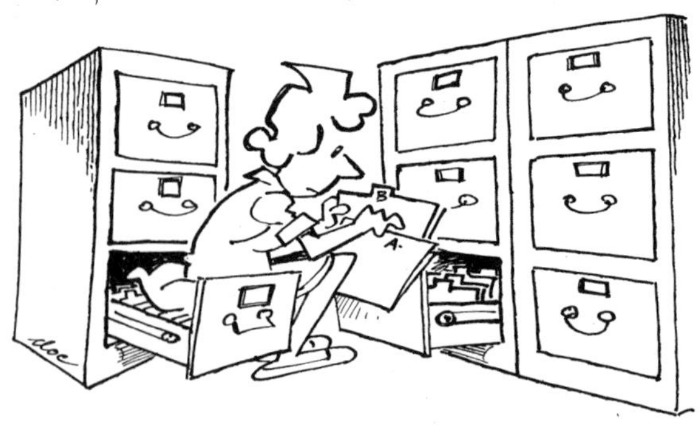

If a nurse or therapist asks you to do something you haven't done, or if it has been a long time since you've done it, be sure you say so. Do not ever be afraid to say you need to review a procedure, for example, a Hoyer lift transfer. Patient safety is a big responsibility, and it is a big part of your responsibility.

Aides may want to make suggestions for educational in-service. Remember that the only "dumb" question is the one that doesn't get asked. It may be that others want the answer to the same question, so speak up!

All certificates for completed continuing education are kept in your personnel or human resource file. For your own records, always keep a copy of the health and continuing education requirements listed below in a safe place. You may receive a request to report for annual or other updates concerning:

- CPR – Cardiopulmonary Resuscitation Certification
- OSHA, standard precautions/blood-borne pathogens
- Safety inservices
- TB Testing – Mantuox skin test or chest x-ray for tuberculosis screening
- Any certificates from in-services you attend on your own
- Annual (or when required) physical exam
- Hepatitis B vaccine status
- Updated immigration information
- Automobile insurance and driver's license information
- Criminal background checks may be required by the state organization
- Other requests for education and files as per your organization employer or specific state or other requirements

These requirements are very important for the smooth operations of your organization. As a career home health aide, it is your responsibility to assure that the needed information is obtained and provided timely to your supervisor or other designated individuals.

Being knowledgeable and responsible for and about your work contributes to increased confidence. This confidence will also be noticed by your patients and give them added security and peace of mind while they are in your care.

DRESSING FOR SUCCESS IN HOME CARE: PUTTING YOUR BEST FOOT FORWARD

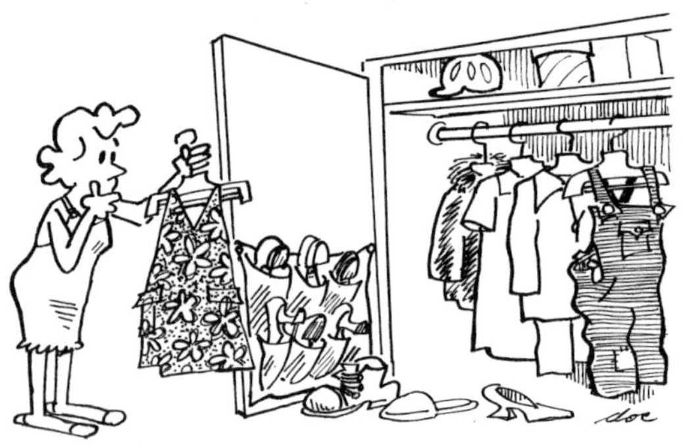

As a team member of your employer or organization, it is your responsibility to be neat, clean, and in uniform, as instructed by the organization's policy. Some organizations require a specific type of uniform, lab coat, or specific colors that are to be worn. These policies are to protect clients and also to protect the staff. Uniforms help clients and families recognize home health care or hospice staff. Your work clothing should be washed as soon as possible after soiling. Never wear open toed shoes (sandals or flip-flops). These can expose your skin to splinters and cuts. Your hair should be neat and away from your face. If your hair is long, it should be tied back.

When you look professional, you are treated that way. No perfume or jewelry should be worn. Perfume can be too strong or cause breathing difficulty for some patients (e.g. COPD, etc.) and nausea for others. Rings and bracelets must not be worn as they can accidentally cause injury to patients. A wedding ring is usually acceptable and only earrings that fit close to or directly on the ear (like small post pearls). Nail polish must be removed or reapplied when chipped. Wear your I.D. pin or name tag according to your organization's policies.

SUMMARY

Assuming responsibility for updating your files and maintaining a neat appearance demonstrates to others that you care about how others see you. It also shows that you strive to do your best for yourself, your patients, and your organization. Always remember that you are a guest in your patient's home and that you represent your organization in the community. Represent them and yourself well!

REVIEW EXERCISES

1) List the in-service training requirements for your position (or other requirements per role and organization). (See page 82).
2) Check with your supervisor to make sure that your personnel file and needed medical and other information is up-to-date. (See page 83)
3) Review your agency's dress code to see if you are following it correctly. (See page 84-85).
4) Identify six to twelve inservices that you have attended in the past year.
5) Describe a topic that you would like to attend an in-service about.

CHAPTER TEN

SAFETY FIRST: HOMEMAKING AND HOUSE-KEEPING CONSIDERATIONS

Depending on your assignment and your patient, you may have homemaking responsibilities. Part of the work of home health care is trying to optimize patient safety --when possible and patients allow us to! According to the Home Safety Council home accidents cause 20 thousand deaths in the United States annually. Many of our frail or elder patients can no longer maintain their homes as they once were able. A clean and tidy home and "patient area" is very helpful for providing care and contributes to patient's feeling better. Important home-making tasks may include meal preparation, laundry, light housekeeping, and other duties that help the patient to remain at home safely. The goal here is patient comfort and safety. For example, if you walk up to the house and see newspapers lying outside on the driveway, pick them up and carry them into the house. If you see food spoiling in the refrigerator, ask the patient about this and offer to throw out the spoiled items and wipe out the refrigerator. Sweeping the kitchen floor or wiping up a spill are both examples of homemaking that support patient safety and comfort. Similarly, if you see clothes that need to be picked up, washed, or folded - - this is something you would do - - it all depends on the aide assignment your supervisor gave you.

If you have a case where the patient is in an unsafe environment, such as where there are numerous animals with no or poor care and animal feces in the home, or there is a hole in the floor, these would be examples of where you should call your supervisor. These examples may need the skills of a social worker and a heavy duty house cleaning service to get the home environment to a level (once cleaned and stabilized) where the patient is safe and the home care team can provide care. Your supervisor may also call in the physical or occupational therapist for home safety assessment. These professionals may also recommend safety equipment such as grab bars and handrails.

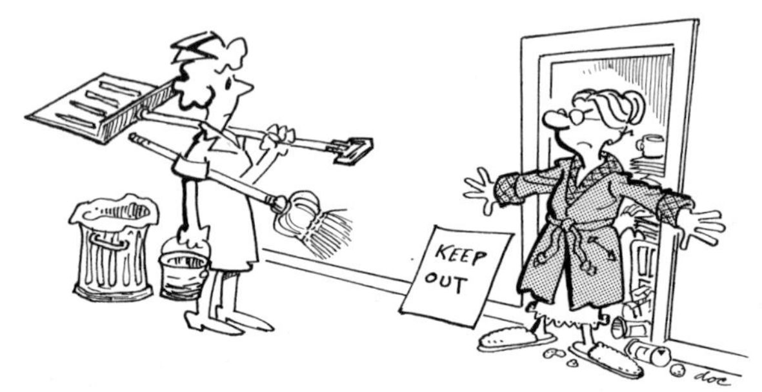

HOUSEKEEPING 101: IMPORTANT SUPPORT FOR PATIENTS TO REMAIN SAFELY AT HOME

Home health aides may also provide some level of housekeeping when meeting the goal of maintaining the environment for home health care. Think about how good it feels when you walk in the door to your home and it looks tidy and clean. Our patients want the same thing - - and you can contribute to this good feeling. For example, when bathing a patient, the aide puts the soiled washcloths and towels in the washer and may start the washer and/or dry the clothes. Similarly you may prepare breakfast for an older adult patient with diabetes and would clean up the dishes after the meal preparation and breakfast activities are completed. Remember that the kitchen and bathroom are considered the most dangerous rooms in any home. If you cook for your patient, make sure the potholders are safe and hole-free and the ovens and stove are turned off when finished with meal preparations and before you leave the patient's home. Remember to always check the temperature of hot water before you or your patient uses it. Your patient, such as patients with diabetes, may have diminished sensation and be burned.

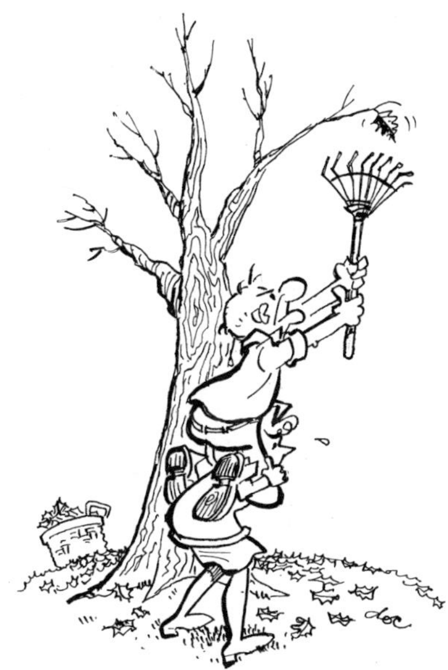

OTHER SAFETY CONSIDERATIONS

Safety considerations when performing housekeeping/cleaning duties include the following:

- Do not use bleach unless directed by the patient, your employer, or your supervisor - - even then, use very carefully.
- Never mix household cleaning products together - - this can cause dangerous fumes!
- Remember that cleaning supplies that have a strong clean odor or smell may be dangerous to some patients - - especially those with asthma, COPD, and other known lung problems. These are the same

patients who should not be around powder or perfume - - check with your supervisor when in doubt. Air out the house, open a window if possible, and do not use caustic and/or strong smelling products around these patients.

- If you clean up the floor after a spill, remember that some cleaners/cleaning products make surfaces – like the floor – shiny and slippery. Be careful and check that the floor is not slippery for you and your patient. You may want to check after cleaning while wearing socks. This simple test would show you if the floor is slippery and unsafe. This includes wood, tile, and marble floors, such as those in a bathroom. The "shine" can be very slippery and dangerous - - remember, safety first!

SUMMARY

Aides in home health or hospice care may find wide variations in the homes that they visit. Your supervisor looks to you for reporting obviously unsafe situations. Housekeeping and homemaking duties are frequently a part of the aide assignment sheet. These simple tasks may often make the difference between a patient being able to remain at home or being sent to a nursing home or the hospital.

REVIEW EXERCISES

1) List three homemaking or housekeeping duties that may be on the aide care plan (See page 87).
2) Describe two unsafe home environments and explain why you would call your supervisor (See page 87-88).
3) Explain the statement: "The kitchen and bathroom are the most dangerous rooms in the house" (See page 88-89).

PART TWO

SPECIAL PATIENT POPULATIONS: GUIDELINES FOR CARE

AIDS (ACQUIRED IMMUNE DEFICIENCY SYNDROME) CARE

1) AIDS Care: AIDS (Acquired Immune Deficiency Syndrome) is a disease that causes the immune system to no longer work effectively. AIDS patients range in age from infancy through the elderly. Patients with AIDS are at risk for all kinds of infections, some of them life-threatening, because their immune response cannot fight the infection. HIV stands for Human Immunodeficiency Virus. HIV is not AIDS but may be seen as a precursor or related illness. HIV is transmitted through high-risk behaviors or other encounters with the virus. The Center for Disease Control has determined that HIV does not survive well in the environment, that is it can easily be killed with soap and water, bleach and water, or sunlight. HIV is carried in blood and semen and can infect an individual if it enters the body or blood stream.

2) General Information: AIDS can be a chronic life-limiting illness characterized by infections and debilitation. Patients with AIDS may face many problems including: pneumonia, diarrhea, shortness of breath, cancer, and weight loss. It is important to maintain standard precautions with all patients, including patients with AIDS, to protect them from any infections. See "Bedbound Care" if appropriate.

3) Home Health Aide Goals of Care:
- Patient clean, safe and comfortable
- Safe assistance with activities of daily living
- Patient assisted with mobility
- Energy conservation
- Infection control measures maintained
- Support to patient
- Patient lifestyle and choices respected throughout care

- Meals of choice prepared and served to patient
- Other goals

4) Personal Care Considerations: Many patients with AIDS are young and were active until they became sick with the infections from AIDS. Give the patient choices about their care regimen. For example, do they want to start with a bath or a meal? Many patients will try and "save" their energy for something important to them, so support that choice.

Patients with AIDS are active members of the health care team. Some patients may need rest periods between activities. Stop if your patient is getting short of breath, and allow the patient time to rest. Ask your patients to let you know when they are ready to continue. Personal care items in these cases must never be shared.

As for all patients and care, explain what you are going to do and what you are doing as you do it.

5) Safety Considerations: Some patients with AIDS are weak. It is important that the aide assist with walking, as necessary. Offer to help your patients. The occupational therapist may be appropriate for an assessment and teaching related to energy conservation and adaptive devices for performing ADLs.

In preparing meals, ask the nurse what the patient may or may not eat. Raw eggs should not be used in meals for patients with AIDS. This is because patients are susceptible to infections from microorganisms, found in eggs.

Patients with AIDS should not change their cat's kitty litter or clean the birdcage. This is also because they are susceptible to infections from microorganisms because of their immune status.

Maintain standard and other precautions as directed by your supervisor. AIDS patients often take many medications. The aide should make note if the aide knows what is being taken.

6) Documentation Tips: Write the care you provide on the aide form. Remember, if the nurse orders a service on the care plan and there is no spot on the aide checklist for that task, write it in longhand on the form under "other." Document coordination of care activities.

7) Special Considerations: Some patients with AIDS are sad and depressed, as they may have lost friends or lovers to the disease. Signs of depression can include crying, sadness, not eating, or a change in sleeping habits among others. If you believe your patient is depressed, let your supervisor know your concerns.

Generally, patients with AIDS need a high calorie and high protein diet to help them replace lost muscle tissue. Increased fluids will help prevent dehydration which is common with a poor appetite, weight loss, diarrhea, and vomiting. Ask the nurse or the dietitian for specific instructions for your patient.

A complex medication regimen is usual for patients with AIDS. The patient may feel the medications are not "useful" or may want to stop taking them since there are often so many. This change may be a sign of depression and the aide should contact the supervisor immediately.

ALZHEIMER'S DISEASE AND DEMENTIA CARE

1) Alzheimer's Disease and Dementia Care:
Alzheimer's Disease is a dementia or progressive decline in cognitive function characterized by confusion, increasing memory loss, disorientation, loss of problem solving abilities, gradual deterioration in ability to function and care for themselves safely, and other problems.

According to the National Institute on Aging, Alzheimer's Disease alone currently affects over four and a half million Americans. President Reagan was one of its victims. Many patients are confused or demented for a variety of reasons, but patients with Alzheimer's Disease eventually begin a functional decline. This means they lose the ability to care for themselves and are unable to feed or toilet themselves and become bedbound.

2) General Information: The difficulty with Alzheimer's and other dementias is the stress on the caregiver(s) and the safety concerns related to caring for confused or disoriented patients. The patient may forget to eat, have difficulty sleeping, or have routines that are difficult for the family or caregivers to address. Safety, health maintenance, prevention of wandering, and support are major roles of the home care organization. There may be a specialized training program for aides and other caregivers about working with patients who suffer from Alzheimer's disease and/or dementia.

3) Home Health Aide Goals of Care:
- Patient clean, safe, comfortable, groomed
- Encourage/support communication
- Safe assistance with activities of daily living
- Patient assisted with and maintains mobility/exercise program
- Caregiver(s) provided support

- Infection control measures maintained
- Patient eats prepared and served meals
- Medication Compliance
- Other goals

4) Personal Care Considerations: Check the temperature of the bath water, as the patient may forget to check these seemingly second-nature safety tasks. Be patient. Understand that some confused patients develop or have a fear of water while some patients with dementia find bathing soothing. The bathing process can be quite scary for some patients, they may be cold and frightened when undressed. Ask your supervisor for assistance with bathing techniques.

Allow the patient to do as much personal and self-care as safely possible.

Try to find out (or establish) the patient's routine, so you can provide personal care in this same way, if possible. Alzheimer's patients do well with strict and consistent routines. You may need to "cue" the patient for the order of desired activities.

As for all patients and care, explain what you are going to do and what you are doing as you do it. Arguing with these patients regarding orientation or how to do things may cause agitation and should be avoided.

5) Safety Considerations: Scan the patient area for any objects that could cause injury to the patient and remove them if possible. Some patients with Alzheimer's and other dementias "wander away" from home. Do not let the patient out of your sight, whenever possible. Keep doors locked and promote the patient's safety, where possible. This may include the family having the gas stove and/or disposal permanently turned off.

The patient might need to be reminded to eat, drink, or urinate. You may be asked to keep track of the patient's intake and output, particularly bowel movements to prevent constipation.

6) Documentation Tips: Write the care you provided on the aide form. Remember, if the nurse orders a service on the care plan and there is no spot on the aide checklist for that task, write it longhand on the form under "other."

7) Special Considerations: When caring for a patient with Alzheimer's, try to also support the spouse, daughter, son, or other caregivers while you are there. Caregiving can be quite stressful. These individuals may need some restful time away.

Sometimes, the AD patient can become agitated for no apparent reason (they may not know where they are or could be asking for their parents). A backrub or gentle foot massage may be helpful to diminish their fear. Try playing "their favorite" music softly.

Remember that the patient and or families are not only losing their loved one as they knew him or her but during the disease process, they also lose their memories. It is very difficult not to be remembered or share in memories.

Generally, a high calorie diet can help to prevent weight loss even if the patient is overweight at this time. Use of simple one step instructions to encourage food intake is helpful to the patient. For example, "Put the food on your fork. Put the food in your mouth. Chew. Swallow." Some patients may find it easier to eat finger foods. Talk with the nursing supervisor about the possible need for a dietitian or nutritionist to see the patient. This is particularly important when your patient has trouble swallowing or has no appetite.

AMPUTATION CARE

1) Amputation Care: Patients may have an amputation due to a disease, such as diabetes, or an infection, such as gangrene, or due to a traumatic injury, such as a motorcycle or car accident.

2) General Information: The loss of a limb is an emotional and traumatic incident in any patient's life. Things we take for granted, like running to answer the phone or getting up to go to the bathroom at night, are altered forever when a patient has to put on a prosthesis to even stand safely. The same loss is true with the upper extremity, the loss of an arm or a hand. It is important that the aide be understanding about the loss and allow patients to do as much as safely as possible for themselves. Sometimes the patient may complain of "phantom pain" in the missing limb. They are called this because even though the leg or arm is gone, the pain and other sensations continue in the missing limb. Report these sensations or other pains or changes to the nurse. Balance can also be difficult after an amputation.

3) Home Health Aide Goals of Care:
- Patient clean, safe and comfortable
- Safe assistance with activities of daily living
- Patient assisted with and has increased mobility
- Infection control measures maintained
- Telephone kept nearby
- Skin integrity maintained/protected in relation to prosthesis attachment areas
- Other goals

4) Personal Care Considerations: It is important to maintain the patient's balance while performing personal care. An example is the patient who uses crutches or a wheelchair, prior to the prosthesis being fitted. Allow the patient time to get safely comfortable. Be aware that a regular wheelchair is not balanced for an amputee and could tip over with reaching or doing ADLs. This is especially true for elderly patients who may take a little more time to adjust to the change and the use of crutches or a prosthesis. Usually, the prosthesis itself should not get wet. Ask the patient, nurse, physical therapist, or occupational therapist about the particular care and safety tips related to the prosthesis.

As for all patients and care, explain what you are going to do and what you are doing as you do it.

5) Safety Considerations: It is very important for the aide to take care of the patient's prosthesis and handle it gently. Prosthetic arms and legs are very costly. Patients would be further severely handicapped in any activity if something happened to their prosthesis.

Be aware that during the adjustment period to a prosthesis, the patient may experience pain, discomfort, and even skin problems such as sores or blisters. If this happens to your patient, any skin problems or changes must be reported immediately to the nurse or therapist.

6) Documentation Tips: Write the care you provided on the aide form. Remember, if the nurse orders a service on the care plan and there is no spot on the aide checklist for that task, write it longhand on the form under "other."

7) Special Considerations: Patients will grieve for the loss of a limb the same as a person grieves for the loss of a loved one. Support the patient and allow this grieving process and be a good listener.

ARTHRITIS CARE

1) Arthritis Care: Arthritis is a condition of inflammation of the joints and is characterized by pain and swelling. It often affects joints in the hands, knees, and hips but can affect many other joints. Although arthritis is primarily seen in older patients, children and young adults can also have arthritis. Refer to the "Pain Management Care" guideline for more in-depth information.

2) General Information: Though there are different kinds of arthritis, such as rheumatoid or osteoarthritis, they all result in pain which causes the patient to move slowly and have decreased range of motion and strength. For the aide this means that positioning or assisting with walking must be done gently and slowly, while allowing the patient to do as much safely and comfortably as possible. These patients generally move more slowly in the early morning due to stiffness and improve somewhat throughout the day.

3) Home Health Aide Goals of Care:
- Patient clean, safe and comfortable
- Joints maintained in functional position
- Function maintained through range of motion (ROM)
- Safe assistance with activities of daily living
- Infection control measures maintained
- Medication compliance
- Energy conservation
- Prevent further complications
- Other goals

4) Personal Care Considerations: Allow ample time for bathing and other personal care tasks.

Keep joints in comfortable and functional positions when moving the patient.

As for all patients and care, explain what you are going to do and what you are doing as you do it.

5) Safety Considerations: Many patients with arthritis are on medications to help their inflammation, swelling, and pain. Know what your patient's usual level of pain is on the pain scale, 0-10. If your patient is having more pain than usual, or complains of pain generally, talk to the nurse. The nurse may want to re-evaluate the patient and talk to the physician about medication or other pain relief measures.

Try to support the patient's safe independence, wherever possible. For example, open jars and make sure that medication bottles are not closed so tightly that the patient cannot move the top (if there are not any children or others who may mistakenly take the medications). These gestures show thoughtful planning which allows patients to remain home independently.

You may be asked to gently perform range of motion exercises. Check with the nurse or therapist about the exercises. If you are not sure how to do them, ask the nurse or therapist for instruction or a demonstration. You may be asked to remind the patient to take ordered medications prior to therapy visits for comfort and so exercises can be performed.

The patient may use ice or heat in addition to medication for pain relief. Assist the patient in using these methods being careful to have a layer of cloth between the heat or ice and the skin. Check the heat temperature to be sure the skin will not be burned. If you notice the cord is frayed, let the nurse or your supervisor know.

6) Documentation Tips: Write the care you provided on the aide form.

Remember, if the nurse orders a service on the care plan and there is no spot on the aide checklist for that task, write it longhand on the form under "other."

Coordinate care when changes occur.

7) **Special Considerations:**

____

____

____

BEDBOUND CARE (CARE OF THE BEDRIDDEN PATIENT)

1) Bedbound Care: Patients who are bedridden or "bedbound" have special problems and needs. Being immobilized causes problems and changes to all the body systems. Bed and chairbound individuals and those unable to reposition themselves should be assessed for other factors which increase the risk for developing pressure ulcers. These factors include immobility, incontinence, nutritional factors including an inadequate dietary intake and impaired nutritional status, and an altered level of consciousness. Please refer to "Pressure Ulcer Care" or other specific patient problems for a more in-depth discussion of these possible patient care needs.

2) General Information: The biggest risk to bedbound patients are bedsores, also called pressure or, as they used to be called, decubitus ulcers. Home health aides have seen many of these. It is important to know that in many cases these can be prevented. A pressure ulcer is any skin lesion caused by unrelieved pressure resulting in damage of underlying tissue. Pressure ulcers usually occur over bony prominences. We have all heard the old nursing saying: "Prevention is the best treatment for bedsores." Proper nutrition and frequent patient positioning changes can contribute to healthy, intact skin. Constipating is another complication of immobility. Bedbound patients also are at risk for lung infections, such as pneumonia. Ask the nurse about encouraging deep breathing and coughing, when possible.

3) Home Health Aide Goals of Care:
- Patient clean, safe and comfortable
- Patient repositioned safely and frequently as designed on plan of care
- Skin problems minimized through care

- Care taken to minimize the force and friction applied to the skin
- Infection control measures maintained
- Bed linens clean, dry, and comfortable
- Bowel protocol monitored and maintained
- Function maintained through ROM (Range of Motion)
- Prevent further complications
- Other goals

4) Personal Care Considerations: Some bedbound patients have indwelling urinary catheters and may be incontinent with their bowels. Meticulous skin care is important in maintaining skin which is free of breakdowns or reddened areas. Encourage the use of ordered skin protector creams. Dense foam, air mattresses, or other systems are commonly used to help prevent pressure areas and may provide comfort for the bedbound patient.

If your patient is incontinent, cleanse skin with mild soap and water and rinse where possible, at the time of soiling. When moisture cannot be controlled, such as with urinary incontinence, use underpads or briefs that are absorbent and present a quick-drying surface to the skin.

The patient's bedbath is an important part of the patient's total care for maintaining hygiene and in keeping the patient clean and comfortable. Allow the patient to have input into their bath routine, as much as possible. Avoid hot water. Use moisturizers for dry skin (with supervisor's permission). The bedbath is also an opportunity to assess the patient's skin and status and to show caring through gentle touch. Use proper positioning, transferring, and turning techniques. Bedbound patients are at risk for "foot drop". Ask your supervisor for special positioning, equipment, or supportive devices such as footboard or bed cradle to prevent this problem. Wearing tennis shoes may also help some patients.

As for all patients and care, explain what you are going to do and what you are doing as you do it.

5) **Safety Considerations:** Be aware of the temperature of the water as the patient may be very sensitive to heat and cold. Wash your hands with warm water before touching the patient. Make sure the personal emergency response system (PERS), if available, is nearby. Fall safety is a major consideration for these patients as well.

Adhere to your organization's policies. Use gloves, and follow standard precautions for personal care if appropriate.

6) **Documentation Tips:** Write the care you provided on the aide form.

Remember, if the nurse orders a service on the care plan and there is no spot on the aide checklist for that task, write it in longhand on the form under "other."

It is helpful to note the number of wet underpads or absorbent briefs, or the amount of urine in the drainage bag, and note bowel movements in the same way on the form. Some programs have a calendar or day sheet that stay in the home, on which this information is entered. In this way, all caregivers have this information when they make visits.

Check with your nurse for any questions you may have. Notify the nurse if you note any reddened areas or other changes.

7) **Special Considerations:** Nutrition and hydration are very important to the maintenance of all body systems, particularly the skin. Follow the HHA assignment sheet related to offering fluid or dietary supplements.

BONE/FRACTURE/JOINT REPLACEMENT CARE

1) Bone/Fracture/Joint Replacement Care: Fractures often occur as a result of falls in older adults because there is a reduction in bone mass that results with aging. Sometimes the bone breaks by itself (a pathological fracture) which causes the fall. Degenerative arthritis or other diseases can cause joint pain in older adults that leads to joint replacement surgery. Many patients are referred to home health care for recovery after hip surgery.

2) General Information: A fall that results in a fracture is a traumatic incident for patients. The fall may sometimes be the reason family members believe that "it isn't safe for Grandma to live alone anymore." It is for this reason that safety in the home, particularly falls precautions, is so important and stressed so frequently as a way to maintain patients independently at home. These patients at first may use an assistive device (walker, cane, quad cane) and they may have been ordered not to put their full weight on the side of the fracture until it is fully healed. They also may have pain when trying to walk and performing their ordered exercises. Notify the nurse if the pain medication appears not to be effective. Osteoporosis, a thinning of the bone mass, also contributes to fractures. Frail, elderly women often have osteoporosis and their posture may be an indication of this disease.

3) Home Health Aide Goals of Care:
- Patient clean, safe and comfortable
- Patient area clean and tidy
- Hip precaution guidelines maintained
- Assistance with home exercise program, after instruction by PT or RN

- Safe assistance with activities of daily living
- Infection control measures maintained
- Nutrition and hydration maintained
- Patient assisted with and has increasing mobility
- Other goals

4) Personal Care Considerations: Patients who are able to wash their upper body should be encouraged to continue to do so, but may need assistance with their lower extremities and other parts of their bath.

Because the patient's incision should be healing, if you observe redness, drainage, or swelling, or the patient complains of pain, report these symptoms immediately to the nurse.

There will be limits in the patient's range of motion on the affected side. The physical therapist may show you how to help the patient perform exercises during personal care.

The patient at first may need to have a bedbath until it is once again safe to have a tub bath or shower. The nurse or therapist will tell you when to change the bath order, based on the patient's progress. An occupational or physical therapist may also be involved in the care and assist with ordered needed assistive or adaptive equipment related to personal care or other activities.

Patients may have a plastic "toilet" or raised toilet seat which sits on top of their own toilet seat. This allows patients to not have to bend unnecessarily when getting on and off the toilet. If your patient has one of these, make sure it is secure before the patient sits down. Keep it clean after use.

As for all patients and care, explain what you are going to do and what you are doing as you do it.

5) Safety Considerations: It is very important for patients to use their assistive device and only put weight on the affected side when, and if, ordered by their doctor.

Be sure the walker or cane is next to the patient at all times, especially when you leave. Also, when possible, leave the phone near the patient for safety reasons. Report any equipment that needs repair to your supervisor.

Only assist the patient with exercises you have been shown how to do by the nurse or therapist.

Be aware that pain or other medications sometimes may make the patient sleepy. Recognize that some medications may increase the risk for falls.

Clear and unclutter path or walkways, if possible. Make sure any liquid spills are completely cleaned or mopped up and dried to prevent slips or tripping.

For safety reasons, make sure lighting is adequate. Remove throw rugs and/or newspapers on floors (with patient/family's permission).

Your patient may need to take pain medication before ADLs are performed, like bathing, so that activity will be more productive and the patient will be more comfortable. The nurse or therapist will tell you this information.

Physical therapy teaches the use of assistive devices such as a cane or walker, while the patient is gaining strength to improve their balance. Occupational therapy assists with compensatory techniques and the use of assistive devices and skills that will help with safe showering or dressing.

6) Documentation Tips: Write the care you provided on the aide form.

Remember, if the nurse orders a service on the care plan and there is no spot on the aide checklist for that task, write it in longhand on the form under "other".

Document any coordination of care information or activities.

7) **Special Considerations:**

BRAIN TUMOR CARE

1) Brain Tumor Care: There are different types of brain tumors. Some are malignant or cancerous and others are benign or not cancerous. Either way, patients with brain tumors admitted to home care may need care after brain surgery, chemotherapy, and/or radiation therapy. Both children and adults can have brain tumors and possibly need care at home, depending on their unique condition and circumstances.

Please refer to "Bedbound Care", "Cancer Care", or "Hospice Care" or other specific patient problems for a more in-depth discussion of these possible patient care needs.

2) General Information: Patients with brain tumors can either be in a home care or a hospice program, depending on the patient's prognosis (how the patient will probably do), the patient's doctor, and the patient and family's wishes. Sometimes brain tumor patients will have intravenous (IV) medications and fluids at home. These patients have been referred to the nursing organization for assistance with the IV and other nursing care. Support for both the patient and their family is also needed.

Sometimes patients with brain tumors can have seizures, also called convulsions. Special care is needed for patients who could have seizures. Ask the nurse to note the symptoms, seizure precautions, and care on your care plan and note this in a home care folder placed in the home.

Your patient may also benefit from the occupational, physical therapist, or speech-language pathologist as he/she may have muscle weakness, balance problems, coordination changes, cognitive and perceptual changes, and/or problems with activities of daily living (ADLs). They may also have problems swallowing or eating and may be referred to a dietitian or nutritionist.

3) Home Health Aide Goals of Care:

- Patient clean, safe and comfortable
- Safe assistance with activities of daily living
- Infection control measures maintained
- Prevention of injury
- Bowel protocol monitored and maintained
- Seizure precautions noted and followed
- Medication compliance
- Patient wishes and requests respected through care
- Other goals

4) Personal Care Consideration: Generally, gentle and supportive care is given to patients at home with a brain tumor.

Many patients with brain tumors are on "steroids", a type of medication that decreases their brain swelling but causes them to appear puffy and have very sensitive skin that may be prone to breakdown. This is one reason that patients who spend time in bed must turn or be helped into varying positions to prevent skin breakdown, such as pressure ulcers.

The patient may have TED or other support hose stockings which must be applied after personal care is completed.

It is important to explain to the patient what you are going to do and allow the patient as much "say" in how the bath and other care are accomplished as safely as possible.

As for all patients and care, explain what you are going to do and what you are doing as you do it.

5) Safety Considerations: Sometimes patients with brain tumors complain of headaches or seizures. If you are present during a seizure, turn the patient on his or her side. The main goal is to protect patients from hurting themselves, such as hitting their heads. In this instance, follow your organization's procedures. After the seizure, call the nurse. The nurse may call the physician about possible medication changes or other changes to the patient's plan of care.

Some patients with brain tumors have balance or walking difficulty. Be sure to leave any assistive devices near the patient to use any devices as ordered.

6) Documentation Tips: Write the care you provided on the aide form.

Remember, if the nurse orders a service on the care plan and there is no spot on the aide checklist for that task, write it in longhand on the form under "other".

If your patient has a seizure while you are present or a seizure is reported by the patient between visits, write the time, what you saw, when you called the nurse, etc. to document your care of the patient.

7) Special Considerations:

____

____

____

BREAST CANCER CARE

1) Breast Cancer Care: The incidence of breast cancer is appropriately alarming to all women. The home care patient with breast cancer also has body image changes with which to cope besides dealing with the cancer diagnosis. It is very important that the HHA be emotionally supportive of the woman with this diagnosis. Please refer to "Cancer Care" and "Hospice Care" or other specific problems for a more in-depth discussion of these patient care needs.

2) General Information: Breast cancer affects both younger and older women. This diagnosis can be particularly difficult for some husbands, boyfriends, or significant others. They may wish to speak with the female team members of the home care staff about their feelings and fears. In addition, a small percentage of men get breast cancer.

3) Home Health Aide Goals of Care:
- Patient clean, safe and comfortable
- Safe assistance with activities of daily living
- Patient's privacy and dignity maintained through care
- Infection control measures maintained
- Assistance with home exercise program
- Bowel protocol monitored and maintained
- Support and patience during the length of care
- Other goals

4) Personal Care Considerations: Privacy can be particularly important for some patients with breast cancer. Be aware that some patients may have difficulty looking at the surgical site and the area of the missing breast.

Be particularly gentle around the patient's chest and surgical area as well as with the patient's arm on the affected side.

Occasionally, machines may be used which help push the swelling out of the arm. They look similar to blood pressure cuffs. Never assist the patient with the use of the machine without the nurse's knowledge and specific instructions and supervision. There may also be a fluid removal system with a drain in the breast (e.g. a hemovac).

As for all patients and care, explain what you are going to do and what you are doing as you do it.

5) Safety Considerations: Ask patients what they want or prefer as you proceed with your care.

As always, explain what you need to do and your assignment duties.

The patient initially may have drains after the surgery. Care must be taken not to pull, tug, or in any way stretch or dislodge the drains. Report any problems to the nurse.

Notify the nurse supervisor of any complaints or changes relating to the wound, pain, or patient complaints or changes which may signify a wound site infection.

Remember **not** to take blood pressures on the arm closest to the mastectomy site. Many times patients experience swelling and pain in that arm, so you need to be particularly careful with it.

6) Documentation Tips: Write the care you provided on the aide form.

Remember, that if the nurse orders it, it needs to be done. If the patient refuses, write that and notify the supervisor, giving the reason if known.

Remember, if the nurse orders a service on the care plan and there is no spot on the aide checklist for that task, write it in longhand on the form under "other".

7) **Special Considerations:** The occupational or physical therapist may also treat your patient due to the pain or limited mobility at the affected site. These rehabilitation team members can also improve the range of motion in the affected upper extremity as well as assist with swelling concerns. Social workers may also be helpful with counseling and a chaplain for spiritual support when available.

CANCER CARE

1) Cancer Care: Many patients are admitted to home care and hospice programs for nursing care due to their cancers. Cancers vary widely, and include blood disorders, such as leukemia, as well as solid tumors, such as lung or stomach "tumors" or growths. Metastases are cancer sites that have spread from the original cancer site. Cancer affects people of all ages, from very young children to the very old.

Please refer to "Brain Tumor Care", "Breast Cancer Care", and "Hospice Care", "Pain Management Care" or other specific problems for a more in-depth discussion of these possible patient care needs.

2) General Information: Patients who have experienced cancer usually have a long history of interaction with members of the health care team. These patients many times are the "experts" on their particular type of cancer and the care they need. It is very important that we listen and provide care based on their individual needs and timetable. Though sometimes difficult, this can make the patient feel better as it allows the patient to have control over his or her care program. Cancer affects the immediate family and the extended family of friends and other caregivers who may be involved with the patient. It is for this reason that we must be particularly sensitive to the needs of patients and their families.

3) Home Health Aide Goals of Care:
- Patient clean, safe and comfortable
- Nutritious meal preparation
- Infection control measures maintained
- Adequate hydration
- Patient comfortable
- Bowel protocol maintained and monitored
- Patient reports feeling clean and comfortable

- Emotional support (patience, kindness) provided to the patient
- Other goals

4) Personal Care Considerations: Patients with cancer may be on powerful medications or "chemotherapy". Chemotherapy may have significant side effects that can make them very tired, lose their hair, bruise easily, be nauseated, vomit, or cause any number of other problems. Monitor pain management for effectiveness.

Radiation therapy, another important treatment for some kinds of cancer, can also cause side effects including general weakness, diarrhea, or skin reactions similar to a bad sunburn in the area being irradiated. Should you see "markings" on the skin, try not to wash them off and do not apply lotions or powders on/to the site. These pen markings are used to identify the specific site for the radiation treatments.

Provide care gently and at the patient's pace. Allow time for the patient to rest between activities.

Be aware and understanding of the loss in self-image related to body changes and hair loss which may occur.

As for all patients and care, explain what you are going to do and what you are doing as you do it.

5) Safety Considerations: A patient with cancer may also have bones which break more easily than usual. Because of this, it is very important to prevent falls and try to create a safe environment for the patient. In fall situations where you would only suffer a sore arm with a black and blue mark, the patient with cancer may have a broken arm from a "pathological" fracture. This means the bone breaks without a fall. Any falls or other problems that you observe during your visit or learn from the patient, should be immediately reported to your supervisor nurse.

6) Documentation Tips: Remember to check off all the items that were assigned to you by your supervisor on the aide assignment sheet or plan.

Remember that the assignment sheet from your supervisor and your documentation form should correspond.

Remember, if the nurse orders a service on the care plan and there is no spot on the checklist for that task, write it in longhand on the form under "other".

7) Special Considerations: Patients with cancer will have varying emotions at the different stages of cancer. Allow patients to discuss feelings and encourage the grieving process for the terminally ill patient and their family.

The occupational or physical therapist may be involved in the care to improve the patient's safe mobility and increase strength as well as for energy conservation.

Patients with cancer may also have a poor appetite. Try to offer snacks of the patient's choice. The organization's dietitian or nutritionist may be called in to assist the patient and increase the intake.

A social worker for counseling or a chaplain for spiritual care may also be involved.

____

____

____

CARDIAC CARE

1) Cardiac Care: Cardiac care patients are patients with heart problems or disease, and have appropriate concerns about their health. Cardiac disease is the leading cause of death in the U.S. Chest pain can be a very scary experience and patients need supportive and gentle care.

2) General Information: Cardiac disease was once considered a "man's disease". However, once a woman passes through menopause, the risk of heart disease increases dramatically. According to the U.S. Department of Health and Human Services, one in five women in the U.S. have some form of cardiovascular or heart disease. The incidence rises to one in three women for age 65 and older.

3) Home Health Aide Goals of Care:
- Patient clean, safe and comfortable
- Patient's wishes and requests respected through care
- Safe assistance with activities of daily living
- Encourage and support independence in self-care
- Infection control measures maintained
- Other goals

4) Personal Care Considerations: Some patients with heart disease will be tired and need frequent rest periods between tasks.

As always, explain what you will be doing before beginning your care responsibilities.

Sometimes you may notice shortness of breath, which may mean the patient is tired and needs a rest between activities. Continue with your duties only after the patient is ready and tells you so.

Some patients will have swelling in their legs or may wear special hose. Many need to keep their legs up as much as possible.

As for all patients and care, explain what you are going to do and what you are doing as you do it.

5) Safety Considerations: Ask the nurse for any special instructions about what to do if your patient experiences chest pain during your care visit.

Some of these patients, particularly if they live alone, may have a personal emergency response system, or PERS, in case they need assistance. If patients have a PERS, they should have it with them at all times. Make sure when you have completed your duties, that the patient is wearing his or her PERS help button.

Many patients with heart conditions are on medicines that can cause dizziness with any sudden movements, such as standing up quickly. Therefore, try to avoid and help them learn to avoid rapid changes in their body position. You may also be asked to check the patient's blood pressure in two different positions (lying down, sitting down, and/or sitting to standing).

Some patients wear patches with medicine to help their heart function. Do not remove these. If the patient needs help applying, be careful not to touch the center where the medicine touches the patient.

The nurse may ask that you weigh the patient every visit. If your patient gains weight, notify your nurse supervisor. This may be a sign of fluid build up and is potentially a very serious condition for patients with cardiac disease.

6) Documentation Tips: The patient's cardio-pulmonary status is very important. Vital signs are important indicators and should be reported to the nurse if outside the parameters or range identified by the nurse.

Document the patient's weight and that you check/take vital signs every visit, or as directed by your supervisor. Also, note any shortness of breath, swelling, chest pain, etc.

Document any coordination of care information.

Write the care you provided on the aide form.

Remember, if the nurse orders a service on the care plan and there is no spot on the aide checklist for that task, write it in longhand on the form under "other".

7) Special Considerations: Some patients with cardiac disease will be using oxygen. Special considerations for nose and throat dryness may need to be taken. Ask your nurse for any recommendations. In addition, the oxygen tubing may also need special care. Ask the nurse for any instructions or duties. Always adhere to your organization's policies about oxygen safety at home. Some patients may also have hospice involved if their heart disease is very severe and what is called "end-stage".

The occupational or physical therapist at your organization may be able to assist your patient with energy conservation techniques which decrease the patient's shortness of breath and pacing activity. Report to your supervisor if there is smoking in the house or the patient uses/has a gas stove or a wood stove. Some patient's may be on nitroglycerin (NTG) pills for their heart. These pills should be left within the patient's reach should they need to take these pills for chest pain. NTG pills go under the patient's tongue to relieve chest pain.

Your cardiac patient may be on a fluid or salt restricted diet. Ask the nurse for any restrictions your patient may have before offering fluids or meals.

CEREBRAL VASCULAR ACCIDENT CARE (CVA/STROKE) AND OTHER NEUROLOGICAL CARE

1) Cerebral Vascular Accident Care: also known as a cerebrovascular accident, a "brain attack", or stroke, is an abnormal condition of the blood vessels in the brain characterized by an embolus, thrombus (blood clots), hemorrhage or bleeding in the brain. These sudden and life-threatening changes result in ischemia (less blood and oxygen flow than normal) which causes less blood circulation to the brain tissues. Strokes are one of the leading causes of death in the U.S.

Strokes can vary widely, based on the extent of the blood flow decrease and the location in the brain. Stroke patients oftentimes have paralysis or weakness, usually on one side, depending on which side of the brain was affected. They can also have speech problems, swallowing problems, and many other problems. They can also be more "emotional" and have changes in their moods. Patients may be depressed, which may also be related to the stroke. Sometimes the patient may cry. As always, if you are concerned, contact the nurse.

Other neurological conditions that may require similar care include Amytrophic Lateral Sclerosis (ALS, also called Lou Gehrig's diseases), Multiple Sclerosis (MS), Parkinson's Disease, and others.

2) General Information: Because of the high frequency of hypertension and other cardiac disease, cerebral vascular accidents, or strokes, continue to be a leading cause of illness, disability, and death. Many patients are admitted to home care after a stroke for continued intensive rehabilitation at home. In these instances, the entire home health care team works in collaboration to assist the patient in meeting goals related to returning to self-care and optimizing rehabilitation.

3) Home Health Aide Goals of Care:

- Patient clean, safe and comfortable
- Affected hands, etc. maintained in functional position
- Patient able to eat and drink safely
- Bowel protocol monitored and maintained
- Communication with patient about care and
  for socialization
- Patient assisted with rehabilitation tasks
- Home exercise program performed
- Application of splints to arms or legs
- Infection control measures maintained
- Observation/reporting related to skin
  problems/pressure from sitting, etc.
- Emotional support related to changes in lifestyle
  caused by the stroke
- Other goals

4) Personal Care Considerations: Have patients involved in as much self-care as safely possible. They may have a routine that they have done for years. If you try to change that routine, it will be harder for patients to return to self-care as they improve in mobility and other areas.

The occupational therapist may assist with equipment to encourage/support independence and to keep the patient safe with ADLs.

As for all patients and care, explain what you are going to do and what you are doing as you do it. The therapist may also be visiting the patient and have safety related or other recommendations.

5) Safety Considerations: The patient who has experienced a stroke may have significant speech and/or swallowing problems that cannot be detected except by experts on the rehabilitation team. For these reasons, speech-language pathologists and occupational therapists may be involved in your patient's care. These specialists may also contribute to the activities on your aide plan of care.

The physical therapist (PT) may provide exercises to the patient to improve leg function, balance, strengthening and mobility. Occupational therapy teaches compensatory techniques and use of assistive devices for safety and maximum independence with ADLs and arm/hand function.

A speech-language pathologist may be involved after the swallowing evaluation is completed to make food recommendations so that the patient does not choke or "aspirate" food or liquids. Aspirate means that food or liquid, "goes down the wrong pipe", the airway instead of the esophagus where food should go, and this may cause aspiration pneumonia. This can occur in stroke patients because the part of the throat which controls this function no longer works. The patient may need to be fed or offered fluids using a straw. Sometimes, a powder is added to liquids to thicken the liquids so it is easier to swallow. Contact your nurse supervisor if you think your patient has a swallowing problem.

Patients may also have "neglect" causing them to forget about the affected side. The patient may be unable to feel hot or cold temperatures with the affected hand so be careful. The patient may not have a shoe on completely or not realize they are lying on their arm. Please be alert to this condition.

If the patient is aphasic, or unable to speak, a personal emergency response system (PERS) should be considered for the patient.

There are two types of aphasia.

Expressive aphasia means the individual understands the written and spoken words but cannot write or speak to communicate clearly.

Receptive aphasia means the individual cannot

understand written or spoken words. Some patients will have both expressive and receptive aphasia, or global aphasia.

Other safety considerations for victims of stroke involve mobility, safe transfer techniques, balance, judgment, and prevention of falls.

6) Documentation Tips: Document the care you provided for the patient on the aide form.

Document any coordination of care information.

Remember that if it is not written, it may appear that it was not accomplished.

Remember, if the nurse orders a service on the care plan and there is no spot on the aide checklist for that task, write it in longhand on the form under "other".

7) Special Considerations:

____

____

____

CHILDREN (CARE OF CHILDREN)

1) Care of Children: It is important to note at the onset that children are different in many ways when they are our patients. In fact, many times the child's mother is the case manager and the primary provider of care. The aide needs to understand normal growth and development for the child's age. Pediatrics or pediatric care means pertaining to preventive and health care treatment of children and childhood diseases and problems. Children may be admitted to home health care or hospice programs for various reasons including: cancers such as leukemia and brain tumors, infusion therapy treatments, infected wounds after surgery, cystic fibrosis, rehabilitation after accidents, and other reasons.

2) General Information: Parents know their child best, so listen to their concerns and recommendations to assist in the child's care. Sometimes you may be caring for the child to give the primary caregiver, usually the mother, a "respite" or break from her all-encompassing 24-hour responsibilities and care. A child's "work" is play, so try to incorporate play into all care routines.

3) Home Health Aide Goals of Care:
- Patient clean, safe and comfortable
- Safely assisted with activities of daily living
- Safe assistance with home exercise program
- Infection control measures maintained
- Patience and kindness
- Other goals

4) Personal Care Considerations: Depending on the child and the child's age, give the child choices about which side to start the bath on, color of washcloth, or soap, toys, or others.

Try to incorporate play whenever possible in the personal care activities.

If you are unsure where to start, ask the child's mother the usual routine and what works best for her child.

As for all patients and care, explain what you are going to do and what you are doing as you do it.

5) Safety Considerations: When caring for infants and children, safety is an important factor to be considered. Safety near windows, poison control, and other safety guidelines should be observed at all times. Crib padding, side rails, toys and other articles should be viewed with child safety in mind.

Sometimes there will be other children, or siblings, who are in the patient's room and may distract you from your tasks.

As a pediatric aide, you may be tested on your specialized skills. You may also have additional training or educational sessions to help you keep current with changes in the pediatric specialty area.

6) Documentation Tips: Write the care you provided on the aide form.

Remember, if the nurse orders a service on the care plan and there is no spot on the aide checklist for that task, write it in longhand on the form under "other".

Document any coordination of care information.

7) Special Considerations:

____

____

____

CHRONIC OBSTRUCTIVE PULMONARY DISEASE (COPD) CARE

1) Chronic Obstructive Pulmonary Disease Care: COPD is a group of lung diseases or problems including emphysema, tuberculosis (TB), asthma, chronic bronchitis, black lung, and other illnesses characterized by breathing problems, respiratory distress, and sometimes the use of oxygen and nebulizer therapies. These are chronic, or long term, in nature.

2) General Information: Patients with COPD are at increased risk for getting respiratory infections. Many of these patients are older adults and have a history of smoking or continue to smoke and may have recurrent episodes of bronchitis or pneumonia.

It is important that patients adhere to their care regimen. These can include many medications, inhalers, oxygen therapy, exercise programs, and "no smoking" orders from their doctor. It is also important that these patients take great care of themselves, adhere to their care program, and avoid infections, which can cause hospitalizations in many cases.

The observations by the aide that the patient's activity tolerance is improving or deteriorating is very important and should be communicated to the nurse.

3) Home Health Aide Goals of Care:
- Patient clean, safe and comfortable
- Bowel protocol monitored and maintained
- Clean air environment maintained (where possible)
- Safe assistance with activities of daily living
- Patient area clean and tidy
- Promote calm environment and reduce stress
- Patient has ordered oxygen on
- Patient can reach telephone/ personal emergency response system

- Assistance with ordered home exercise program
- Infection control measures maintained
- Energy conservation
- Support the patient in stop smoking/cessation efforts
- Other goals

4) Personal Care Considerations: Many patients with COPD or one of the diseases listed above will need frequent rest periods between activities. This includes bathing, eating, walking, and even talking.

The occupational therapist can assist the patient with energy conservation and breathing exercises to minimize shortness of breath (SOB) with activity, to help them remain as active as possible. If you notice your patient is short of breath, allow them to take a break from the activity. Do not change the oxygen flow meter.

As for all patients and care, explain what you are going to do and what you are doing as you do it.

5) Safety Considerations: A physical therapist (PT) or occupational therapist (OT) may help these patients with energy conservation and/or other activities. Always adhere to your organization's policies about oxygen safety. Contact your supervisor if you believe your patient continues to smoke and uses oxygen. This combination causes fires and can result in very serious injury. No candles should be in use or petroleum (like Vaseline) products. Always document if your patient is reluctant to follow oxygen safety precautions.

Oxygen equipment such as nebulizers or concentrators with humidifiers need cleaning regularly. You may be asked to keep the equipment clean. Ask your supervisor about instructions and your role (if any) with home medical equipment cleaning or maintenance.

Be aware of the issue of safety with mobility if the oxygen tubing runs throughout the house; use caution for fall prevention. If your patient has a tracheostomy, which is an opening to breathe in the trachea, near the base of the throat, do not use powder or other products that could cause irritation to the patient. Also avoid perfumes, candles, scented deodorants, etc. If the tracheostomy tube looks loose or the site has other changes, call your supervisor immediately for instructions.

Smoking can also be a major irritant to the delicate tissues surrounding the tracheostomy site and must be avoided. This includes family members and visitors - - contact your nurse supervisor if you experience this problem with your patient.

6) Documentation Tips: Document the care you provided to the patient.

Document what you observe during your visit. Documentation may include that patients are using their oxygen, coughing, experiencing shortness of breath, the doctor makes a home visit, and other objective information that you note that will be communicated about your patient to the supervisor.

Remember, if the nurse orders a service on the care plan and there is no spot on the aide checklist for that task, write it in longhand on the form under "other".

7) Special Considerations: Special considerations may be given for nose and/or throat dryness for patients on oxygen therapy. Ask your supervisor for instruction or recommendations.

These types of patients are often very anxious which sometimes also causes more shortness of breath problems. Try to stay calm with these patients.

Some agencies have policies about patients who have oxygen and continue to smoke. This behavior is unsafe and should be reported immediately. Oxygen supports flame and is absorbed by material (drapes, upholstery) so patients who turn "off" O2 to smoke are not necessarily using safety considerations and you should speak to your supervisor about this immediately.

CHRONIC RENAL FAILURE CARE
(KIDNEY FAILURE)

1) Chronic Renal Failure Care: Chronic renal failure occurs when the kidneys become diseased and are unable to purify the blood of waste products. The body then requires an artificial means (peritoneal, PD, or hemodialysis, HD) to maintain fluid and electrolyte balance. Sometimes this means the patient will have very little urine output. Ask the nurse for specifics about your patient's renal status.

2) General Information: These patients often have had diabetes or hypertension prior to their kidney failure. They are often on multiple medications and have a long history of multiple hospitalizations and doctor visits and frequent home health care intervention.

3) Home Health Aide Goals of Care:
- Patient clean, safe and comfortable
- Patient area clean and tidy
- Infection control measures maintained
- Skin care as instructed by nurse
- Home safety maintained
- Other goals of care

4) Personal Care Considerations: Patients with renal failure often have low endurance or stamina and may need rest periods between tasks.

Your patient may have dry skin and complain of itchiness. Often patients are on medication to reduce the itchiness. Check with the nurse regarding any special skin care. Remind the patient not to scratch and check the patient's fingernails. If the nails are too long, the nurse may assist patients to cut their fingernails.

Patient compliance with dietary/fluid restrictions is important. Ask the nurse or dietitian about your patient's special dietary needs and specific fluid restrictions. You may need to record intake and output on these patients.

Those patients undergoing hemodialysis will have a surgically created access to their veins called a fistula. The fistula makes the veins in that arm or leg very large and prominent. Call the nurse with any problems or changes related to the patient's fistula. **Blood pressures and venipunctures (blood drawing) should never be attempted in the affected arm.** Patients should not carry heavy objects with this arm.

As for all patients and care, explain what you are going to do and what you are doing as you do it.

5) Safety Considerations: Due to the loss of kidney function, many other systems of the body are affected. These patients may:

- Feel colder easily
- Be unable to correctly feel water temperatures (so check for your patient)
- Feel dizzy when standing up and need close supervision when walking
- Feel especially weak after a dialysis treatment

Some patients are treated with peritoneal dialysis, through a small catheter placed in the abdomen, fluid is allowed to flow through large bags of special solution. The solution flows out into another large drainage bag over a specified period of time.

The nurse and/or the patient will care for the catheter at the entry site. The nurse can provide further teaching about this disease and its treatment.

As stated above, blood pressures and venipunctures (blood drawing) should **never** be tried in the affected arm where the fistula or catheter is located.

6) Documentation Tips: Remember that the assignment sheet from your supervisor and your documentation sheet should correspond.

Document any coordination of care.

If the nurse orders a service on the care plan and there is no spot on the aide checklist for that task, write it in longhand on the form under "other".

7) Special Considerations: The patient may be on a kidney transplant waiting list. Ask the nurse about any special instructions related to this status. As with all chronic or long-term illness, your patients and their families also need emotional support.

Your organization may have a dietitian to assist your patient with renal diet and fluid restrictions.

____

____

____

CONSTIPATION CARE

1) Constipation Care: Constipation is the difficulty in passing stools or having bowel movements. Particularly in older adult or bedridden patients, it is thought that functional impairment occurs in the colon, as the patients can no longer respond to the urge to defecate, or have a bowel movement (BM).

2) General Information: There are many factors which contribute to constipation. These include immobility, dehydration, medications, less than optimal bulk and fluid intake, hemorrhoids, chronic use of enemas, and others. Contact the patient's nurse if you notice any symptoms of constipation which include: decreased frequency in bowel movements; hard formed stools; straining; pain while having bowel movement; liquid stools around an impaction; stomach distention (hard, round, big); patients say they feel "full"; uncomfortable, or have no appetite; bleeding with bowel movement; or other changes noted.

3) Home Health Aide Goals of Care:
- Patient clean, safe and comfortable
- Patient repositioned safely
- Bowel protocol monitored and maintained
- Encouraged proper fluid intake and foods high in fiber
- Infection control measures maintained
- Assistance with home exercise program
- Other goals

4) Personal Care Considerations: When providing personal care, particularly to elderly or bedridden patients, keep track of their bowel movements and write this on your HHA documentation form.

During the bath, ask your patients when they had their last bowel movement. If you observe the patients having a bowel movement, document it for size and consistency. In addition, be aware that patients may be constipated and still have leaking diarrhea. Notify the nurse of these symptoms.

If you see external hemorrhoids on your patient, let the nurse know. The patient may need a stool softener or a bowel program to get them back on track and feeling comfortable again. Hemorrhoids can become very inflamed and painful with constipation, which only magnifies the constipation problem.

Hemorrhoids can bleed as hard stool scrapes the area of the hemorrhoid. Notify the nurse if you identify any bleeding after stools. Your patient may need hemorrhoid cream for comfort - - call your nurse for any questions.

As for all patients and care, explain what you are going to do and what you are doing as you do it.

5) Safety Considerations: Older adults can get dehydrated very easily from not drinking enough water, taking certain medication or other reasons. Dehydration contributes to constipation. An intake of increased fluids (unless the patient has fluid restrictions), a diet high in fruit, vegetables, and whole grains can assist with relieving constipation.

6) Documentation Tips: Document the last bowel movement reported to you by the patient or family caregiver.

Document this information on your form and/or on the calendar that remains in the patient's home, depending on your program.

Remember, if the nurse orders a service on the care plan and there is no spot on the aide checklist for that task, write it in longhand on the form under "other".

7) Special Considerations: Nutrition, hydration, medications and dietary habits can contribute to constipation and the right diet can prevent or improve the problem. Encourage your patients to increase intake of fruits and vegetables, and drink plenty of water (unless your supervisor says otherwise due to patient fluid restrictions). A good time to encourage fluid is while you are providing care or preparing and serving meals or snacks.

Exercise, when possible, can also assist in resolving and preventing constipation.

DEPRESSION CARE

1) Depression Care: Depression is a mood disturbance or feeling characterized by sadness, discouragement, and loss. There are many kinds of depression and treatments may include medications, counseling, and other methods, based on the patient's unique needs. The patient's mental health is important and the home health aide can be the person who sees the patient the most and notices a change.

2) General Information: Many of the patients cared for in home care or hospice have appropriate feelings of loss or grief. Illness or sickness itself is a loss of good health. A patient who loses a leg can be very depressed about not being able to do the same activities again, even with a prosthesis. Depression can be a serious problem when patients do not want to eat, get dressed, or care for themselves. If you notice sadness or behavior differences in your patient, such as crying, not wanting to get up or get dressed, notify the nurse. A serious concern is suicide – contact the nurse if you think the patient may be suicidal or seems more depressed.

Remember, many elderly patients lose their life-long spouse, friends, and peers to death or illness. Your organization may have a chaplain, a social worker, or a psychiatric nurse that can help the patient with grief and loss. Because you may be the first or only one to see the depression, your input can be extremely important. Report these observations to the nurse.

3) Home Health Aide Goals of Care:
- Patient clean, safe and comfortable
- Medication compliance
- Patient area clean and tidy
- Assist in identifying stress factors in patient

- Emotional support
- Patient eating and actively participating in ADLs
- Medication compliance
- Infection control measures maintained
- Other goals

4) Personal Care Considerations: When providing personal care, listen to patients and support them through their illness. Some patients "do not want to worry" their spouse and so they may share feelings with you about their loss of good health or mobility. Effective communications, particularly being a therapeutic listener, is very important. For example, it is not appropriate to tell the patient to "Look on the bright side," or "Grin and bear it."

It is very important for patients to take their medications at the prescribed times. Report to the nurse or supervisor those patients who do not take medications as prescribed. Monitor pill boxes for proper use of medications if the aide care plan addresses this.

As for all patients and care, explain what you are going to do and what you are doing as you do it.

5) Safety Considerations: If patients say they want to "give up" or do something to hurt themselves, this is a sign of serious depression and potential suicide. There may be special safety considerations for the potentially suicidal patient that the HHA should be alert to. Ask the nurse supervisor for instructions. Notify the nurse immediately if the patient expresses thoughts of suicide. The nurse may then visit.

Also remember fall safety precautions as these patients may be on numerous medications. The side effects can cause drowsiness and dizziness in some patients.

6) Documentation Tips: Document the care provided on the aide form. Document your communications with your supervisor or the office about your patient.

Remember, if the nurse orders a service on the care plan and there is no spot on the aide checklist for that task, write it in longhand on the form under "other".

Document any coordination of care activities.

 7) **Special Considerations:** Some agencies employ psychiatric nurses who will help patients with depression as well.

____

____

____

DIABETES MELLITUS CARE

1) Diabetes Mellitus Care: Diabetes mellitus is a disorder characterized by a lack of or insufficient insulin. Insulin is very important because it helps the body to utilize sugars or carbohydrates in foods. Diabetes is a chronic disease that usually remains with patients throughout their lives. Children as well as adults can have diabetes mellitus. Treatment is a combination of oral medication or insulin injections, diet, and exercise, depending on the type of diabetes.

Please refer to "Amputation Care" and "Wound Care" or other specific patient problems for a more in-depth discussion of those possible patient care needs.

2) General Information: Diabetes mellitus can be controlled and the long-term effects decreased with lifestyle changes relating to diet and exercise. It is important that patients with diabetes have an established routine of eating at specific times of the day. Patients who take insulin must eat a certain amount of calories each day, as ordered by their doctor. They may have life-threatening problems if they are unable or choose not to eat as required.

Circulation changes may occur with age and may sometimes result in amputations of the lower extremities. As these changes occur, patients may "lose feeling" or sensation in their hands and feet and some may have pain or burning in their lower extremities (this pain is called neuropathy). Other complications of diabetes are poor eyesight or blindness, renal (kidney) problems, and others. Depending upon the type of insulin ordered by the doctor, snacks in the mid-afternoon and before bedtime may be needed.

3) Home Health Aide Goals of Care:

- Patient clean, safe and comfortable
- Skin clean and dry, especially feet
- Infection control measures maintained
- Dietary guidelines supported
- Assistance with meal preparation
- Medication compliance
- Patient area clean and tidy
- Home safety related to vision and circulation changes/problems
- Safe assistance with activities of daily living
- Assist with monitoring blood sugar levels
- Other goals

4) Personal Care Considerations: Patients with diabetes have poor circulation and nerve damage so they may be unable to tell how warm their bath/shower water is. **It is very important to always check the temperature of the water before the patient gets in the tub or shower.**

Patients with diabetes also have decreased circulation and sensation in their feet, so foot care is an important duty that may be part of the care plan. Toe nail care is also very important, however, DO NOT CUT TOENAILS. Due to the poor healing of these patients, a nick caused by cutting a nail may worsen the patient's condition. Usually a podiatrist or other specialist cuts the nails of patients with diabetes mellitus. Always dry between the patient's toes after a foot soak. This is the time to help the patient to examine for skin breaks or other changes which should be reported to the nurse. Ask the nurse about using lotion and a foot rub to increase circulation and to keep the skin supple. The patient **should never ambulate with bare feet.** If patients with diabetes get a sore on their feet, it may be very difficult to heal. In addition, if your patient's feet are swollen, his or her shoes may fit poorly, which may cause rubbing and other skin problems. For this reason it is very important that the patient wear clean and dry white socks that are not too big or too small to cause pressure.

As for all patients and care, explain what you are going to do and what you are doing as you do it.

5) Safety Considerations: It is important to keep patient areas neat and free of any sharp objects that could be stepped on or cause a skin break.

Pathways must be clear and lighting bright enough so patients with decreased vision can get around safely.

The nurse may ask the aide to get "reported" blood sugars each visit and record this information. If a patient's blood sugar drops too low, they may act differently to you. This requires **immediate attention**. Ask the nurse to tell you what to do for each patient if this happens. The patient may be used to this and ask you for some orange juice, which can be used to treat low blood sugar.

6) Documentation Tips: Write the care you provide on the aide form.

Write any special care ordered by the nurse on the care plan if there is not a place on the aide checklist. This could include items such as available food for the patient and whether the patient ate a meal during the aide's visit. Document any coordination of care activities (examples: skin changes, symptoms of low blood sugar, etc).

Remember, if the nurse orders a service on the care plan and there is no spot on the aide checklist for that task, write it in longhand on the form under "other".

Document any coordination of care activities.

7) Special Considerations: If you see any change in your patient with diabetes, call the nurse!

Symptoms of low blood sugar include: perspiration, feeling hungry, feeling lightheaded, tremors, anxiety, weakness, nausea, complaints of nightmares, restless sleep, confusion.

Symptoms of high blood sugar include: increased thirst, fruity breath, increased urination, abdominal pain, nausea, weakness, lethargy, and weight loss.

Because the symptoms are very serious and can be different in various patients, call the nurse with any questions.

If your patient is not eating, or eating foods high in sugar, contact the nurse.

____

____

____

DYING OR END-OF-LIFE CARE

1) Dying or End-of-Life Care: Dying is the process of passing from this physical life. End-of-life care is provided to patients at a time when their illness starts the dying process. This care applies to any person who has an illness which results in death. Treatment and care is directed toward comfort measures and supportive care. The goals of the care at end-of-life (EOL) are relief of uncomfortable symptoms, such as pain or nausea; and comfort interventions, such as hand massages and soft, clean, wrinkle-free sheets. This "palliative" focus promotes comfort.

Please refer also to "Bedbound Care", "Cancer Care", "Hospice Care" or other specific problems for a more in-depth discussion of these patient care needs.

2) General Information: The care of the dying patient is an emotional and difficult time for the patient, as well as for the family and friends. It is important to allow the patient and family to make as many care decisions as they are able. Your caring presence and competent care of the patient may allow them to sometimes take a break. The aide must be very understanding of the difficult times and stress caused by this experience.

3) Home Health Aide Goals of Care:
- Patient clean, safe and comfortable
- Bowel protocol monitored and maintained for patient comfort
- Patient area clean and tidy
- Energy conservation techniques
- Infection control maintained
- Patient's family's wishes and requests respected through care
- Safe assistance with activities of daily living
- Emotional support to patient/family

- Patient and family making as many decisions and maintaining as much control as possible
- Death with dignity
- Other goals

4) Personal Care Considerations: Gentle and supportive care is needed by all patients, but particularly by very sick and dying patients. It is important to move the patient slowly at his or her own pace, to minimize pain or discomfort. There may be days when the patient chooses not to have a bath, or eat breakfast. If the patient is not eating or drinking, mouth care is important as a comfort measure. The aide often must perform all personal care for the patient.

It is important to explain to the patient what you are going to do and allow, as safety permits, the patient to have as much "say" as possible in how the bath or other activity is accomplished.

Skin care is particularly important with patients as they become more bedridden. The patient should be turned to prevent skin breakdown, where possible. The patient and bed linen must be kept clean, dry, and wrinkle-free. The balance between care interventions and comfort for patients is important to consider. If you are unsure about moving or turning a patient, or if moving or turning is painful for the patient, speak to the nurse for direction.

Your patient may appreciate your playing quiet, soft, relaxing music or placing their pet on the bed or near them.

Monitor medications for action(s) and report to the nurse if not working/effective for the patient. As for all patients and care, explain what you are going to do and what you are doing as you do it.

5) Safety Considerations: The patient may have medications being administered by intravenous (IV), subcutaneous lines, or have a "pump". Special care must be given to make sure that these tubes or lines do not become unattached, kinked, or otherwise interrupted. Do not use scissors near the IV and tubing. Patients may also be receiving medications, such as those for pain or nausea relief, which may make transfers and ambulation unsafe. These medications may cause the patient to be groggy or weak. Support your patient with walking and transfers, as it may be unsafe for the patient to do these activities alone. Check with the nurse for specific details of care for these very sick patients and/or for information about the pump.

6) Documentation Tips: Write the care provided on the aide form. Remember, the documentation shows the care you provided to the patient. Complete the form accurately, completely, and legibly.

Remember, if the nurse orders a service on the care plan and there is no spot on the aide checklist for that task, write it in longhand on the form under "other".

Document any coordination of care activities.

7) Special Considerations: Different cultures and families have varied religions and traditions. There are differences in beliefs about life and death. It is very important for the family to be able to uphold or experience their own unique beliefs and traditions, even if they are very different from your own. The aide should support these traditions and follow patient and family wishes about end-of-life care.

The expression of grief or feelings of loss or sadness are also different among families. Sometimes, there may be no expression of grief or grief may be expressed as anger. Talk to your supervisor about any questions you may have while trying to provide the safest and kindest care to your patient.

If family members become hostile with you and/or won't allow you to provide proper care, call your nursing supervisor; do not insist.

If a patient is in home health, your patient may move or transfer to "hospice". Remember this is part of the process and your patient's individual needs may be met better through the hospice program.

STAGES OF GRIEF

Dr. Elisabeth Kubler-Ross was an expert on death and dying issues. She identified five "stages" of grief[1]. It is important to note that all patients have their own unique responses. The aide and other caregivers must support the patient and family through each stage of the dying process. Keep in mind that the stages do not always occur in this order or may appear to occur together. The stages and supportive responses are:

1. Denial - This stage occurs usually after the initial diagnosis and the patient responds with shock and denial due to the awareness and knowledge of the fatal or terminal illness.
   Intervention/Care - Patience and willingness to talk are important at this stage.

2. Anger - This stage usually follows denial. Patients are appropriately angry and ask "why me?" at this stage as well as during various stages throughout the process.
   Intervention/Care - Treat the patient with understanding and respect, do not return the anger.

3. Bargaining - Bargaining occurs when the patient attempts to postpone the illness and death.
   Intervention/Care - If the "bargain" is revealed, listen.

4. Depression - Depression is a part of the dying and grieving process. Patients have many things to grieve over, including hair loss, loss of strength and their prior activity level, loss of health, anticipating future losses, and many others, as unique as the patient and the kind of health problem.

Intervention/Care - Allow the patient to express him/herself fully.

5. Acceptance - Acceptance is the final stage of dying. In this stage, the patient is no longer angry or depressed but has accepted that death is inevitable. Some patients reach a peaceful plateau at this stage.

Intervention/Care - There is no need to encourage talking or activity, simply being with the patient is enough.

[1] Kubler-Ross, E: *On Death and Dying,*
New York, Scribner Publishing Co., 1997.

GASTROSTOMY/JEJUNOSTOMY TUBE CARE

1) Gastrostomy/Jejunostomy Care: A gastrostomy is a surgically-made opening in the abdomen through which a tube is inserted into the stomach. Through this tube a patient receives liquid nutrition and/or medications. This process is performed on patients who cannot ingest, chew, or swallow normal food for a variety of reasons. These reasons include throat or esophageal cancer, CVA (stroke), or the patient who is expected to be unconscious (comatose) for a long period of time.

2) General Information: The change in the way nourishment is achieved from chewing to pouring through a tube can be very upsetting to the alert patient with a gastrostomy (G-tube). Patients may miss the act of tasting food and the socialization that goes along with family meals. The patient and family members may be embarrassed or uncomfortable about seeing the administrations of the feedings.

3) Home Health Aide Goals of Care:
- Patient clean, safe and comfortable
- Bowel regime monitored and maintained
- Safe assistance with activities of daily living
- Tube site clean and healed
- Infection control measures maintained
- Emotional support
- Minimized skin problems through care
- Other goals

4) Personal Care Considerations: Patients with gastrostomy tubes may have many personal care needs. The skin around the site should be kept clean and dry. Drainage or feeding leakage or redness at the site should be noted and reported to the nurse Immediately.

As for all patients and care, explain what you are going to do and what you are doing as you do it.

5) Safety Considerations: There should never be tension or pulling on the G-tube itself. The G-tube end should be secured on the abdomen with tape when not in use. The tape should be relocated on the skin each time it is changed. There should be a plug or way to keep the tube clamped when not in use. If the tube should accidentally fall out, the nurse must be notified immediately. The aide should not participate in putting anything into the G-tube. Also, do not use scissors near a G-tube.

Observe the area/skin site where the tube is placed. Report changes/redness, etc. to nurse.

6) Documentation Tips: Write the care you provided on the aide form.

It is helpful to note the number, date, color, and consistency of bowel movements on the aide form.

Remember, if the nurse orders a service on the care plan and there is no spot on the aide checklist for that task, write it in longhand on the form under "other".

7) Special Considerations: If your patient's abdomen feels hard to the touch, notify the nurse, check the last bowel movement and/or for any episodes of diarrhea

HEART FAILURE (HF) CARE

1) Heart Failure (HF) Care: Heart failure is a condition characterized by impaired cardiac (heart) pumping. Please refer to "Cardiac Care" or other specific problems for a more in depth discussion of these possible patient care needs.

2) General Information: Home health care patients with heart failure, particularly older adults, can be short of breath, tire easily, and have swelling of the ankles and legs. Patients are usually on cardiac medications to improve their cardiac efficiency. These drugs should decrease these symptoms. These medications often cause frequent urination.

3) Home Health Aide Goals of Care:
- Patient clean, safe and comfortable
- Patient area clean and tidy
- Bowel protocol monitored and maintained
- Infection control measures maintained
- Energy conservation measures provided
- Assist with safe ambulation
- Other goals

4) Personal Care Considerations: Plan for frequent rest periods when patients are experiencing shortness of breath or need additional time during bathing or other personal care activities.

Many patients with cardiac problems must be weighed regularly. These weights are very important and should be reported in your documentation and in the report to your supervisor. You may be asked to call the nurse in the event of a weight gain.

Some patients who take fluid pills may "leak" urine, so good personal care is essential.

Some patients have swelling in their legs. This swelling may cause the skin to break down. Elevating the legs may help decrease the swelling. The patient's skin and swelling or any change should be checked at each visit. Report to the nurse any changes.

Commodes may be used by these patients to make urination easier. Cleaning/emptying the commode may be part of the aide plan of care.

As for all patients and care, explain what you are going to do and what you are doing as you do it.

5) Safety Considerations: Some cardiac medications can make patients dizzy and feel "woozy". Have your patients, particularly older adult patients, sit on the side of the bed before standing up in the morning or before making any sudden position changes. In addition, when patients have been sitting, have them take their time standing up. This procedure allows their bodies time to adjust to the change in position.

The aide may be asked to take the patient's blood pressure sitting and standing. Expect the standing blood pressure to be decreased. Report any significant change or other concerns, such as dizziness or increased weakness to the nurse.

6) Documentation Tips: Document the care you provided on the aide form.

Write clearly and always put your name, your title, the date, time, and the patient's name in the designated areas for that important information.

Remember, if the nurse orders a service on the care plan and there is no spot on the aide checklist for that task, write it in longhand on the form under "other".

Document any coordination of care information/activities.

7) Special Considerations: For patients on oxygen, special consideration should be given to the dryness of the patient's nose and throat. Ask the nurse for recommendations. These patients may also need oxygen. Adhere to your organization's policies related to oxygen and oxygen safety.

Your cardiac patient may be on a fluid or salt restricted diet. Ask the nurse for any restrictions your patient may be on, before offering fluids or meals.

Sometimes patients are allowed to increase the number of liters (flow of oxygen) during activity.

HOSPICE CARE

1) Hospice Care: Hospice or hospice care is a special way of caring for patients who have a life-threatening illness which focuses on management of pain and other symptoms associated with the patient's diagnosis and the approaching end-of-life. A terminal illness means the same as a limited life expectancy. Patients admitted to hospice can have varying diagnoses. These can include cancer, AIDS, brain tumors, end-stage renal disease, end-stage COPD, Alzheimer's, and heart failure. Both cancer and non-cancer diagnoses are cared for by hospice. See also "Dying or End-of-Life Care".

2) General Information: The hospice aide, sometimes called a certified nursing assistant (CNA), provides a very special and valuable role in the care of hospice patients and their families. Hospice cares for and supports patients, their family, and their friends.

Team members involved in hospice may be the same or different from home care, depending on the scope of the program and the patient's and family's unique needs. Hospice team members include nurses, a spiritual counselor, a bereavement counselor, occupational or physical therapists, social workers, hospice aides or certified nurses assistants, the medical doctor, and other services, based on the unique patient and family needs.

However, hospices also have very specially trained volunteers. Even after the patient's death, hospice support and caring continues with bereavement support for the family. Bereavement is the period of loss or grief after losing a loved one.

The hospice focus is on quality of life. Simply put, hospice supports the patient and family in making every remaining day the best that it can be. This includes physical, spiritual, and emotional support and honoring patient and family wishes.

Hospice care is more of a philosophy than a building or a setting. Most hospice care is provided at home, but patients may also be admitted to the hospital or other inpatient settings for hospice care. Wherever the site of care, patient wishes are honored and symptom management is the key goal of hospice care.

3) Home Health Aide Goals of Care:

- Patient is clean, safe and comfortable
- Patient's (and family's) wishes are respected throughout care
- Patient's quality of life supported
- Patient's wishes honored
- Patient safely assisted with activities of daily living
- Patient area clean and tidy
- Bowel protocol monitored and maintained
- Infection control measures maintained
- Patient area clean and tidy
- Observe/report pain and management
- Support to hospice patient and family
- Energy conservation for patient and family
- Observation and reporting of pain and other symptoms
- Other goals

4) Personal Care Considerations: Because the focus of hospice is caring, patients often make their own choices, whenever safe and possible. For example, they choose what they want to eat, whether they want a bath or shower (depending on how they feel that day), and their activity schedule. In hospice, the family is an active part of the care plan. This means the family may do as much or as little as they are able to do. The primary caregiver, who may be a family member or a friend of the patient, may be exhausted from caring for the patient on a daily basis. The aide in hospice plays an important role in providing a break for the family or caregivers.

Hospice team members are specialists in managing pain and other symptoms of the disease or treatments. An overall goal of hospice is pain management and symptom relief. If you notice your patient has pain, is uncomfortable, or has other problems such as vomiting or constipation, call the nurse. The nurse may speak with the patient's physician to discuss needed changes to the plan of care. Because of the medications used to control pain, constipation may be a problem. The nurse will provide a bowel protocol for each patient to manage this side effect and symptom.

If your hospice patient is bedridden, skin care is very important to prevent pressure ulcers or other problems that will be painful to the patient. Ask the hospice nurse for any tips about skin care for your patient. Special mattresses can also be utilized to increase comfort for your patients.

As for all patients and care, explain what you are going to do and what you are doing as you do it.

5) Safety Considerations: The hospice philosophy emphasizes that patients and families live life fully every day and that every day is a gift. With this in mind, your patient, on good days, will want to be active. This could mean walking outside to their garden, having a special friend over, or whatever your patient enjoys. Assist your patients in these activities, if possible, to help assure their safety.

Sometimes the illness and medications may make your hospice patient feel dizzy and confused. If your patients feel this way when they change position, have them sit on the side of the bed for a few moments, before attempting to stand. Provide support and assist these patients in standing and walking. If this persists, call the office and speak with your supervisor. Do not attempt to transfer or ambulate your patient if he/she is unsteady. Always be aware of fall safety precautions.

Ask your patients how they are doing and what you can do to make your visit better for them. Offering backrubs, turning on their favorite music, bringing their pet in (or putting it outside for them) and other small acts that demonstrate your kindness and understanding of their special needs at this time.

6) Documentation Tips: Document the care you provided on the hospice aide form.

Document on the correct form. Some programs have special forms for hospice patients. Ask your supervisor if you have any questions about the forms.

Document the patient's bowel movements, as constipation can be very uncomfortable and the goal of hospice is to promote comfort. Contact the nurse if this is a problem so it can be addressed and resolved.

Remember, if the nurse orders a service on the care plan and there is no spot on the aide checklist for that task, write it in longhand on the form under "other".

Document any coordination of care activities.

7) Special Considerations: Hospice care is a team approach. The hospice aide is a valuable member of the hospice team. Hospice teams also meet or have care conferences about the patients and discuss their care needs in meetings called "case conferences" or interdisciplinary group (IDG) or interdisciplinary team (IDT) meetings. You may be asked to attend meetings about your patients. This is also the time to ask the nurse or to her team members questions you may have about improving your care and the patient's comfort. Some hospices involve the hospice aide in "continuous quality improvement" meetings or processes, staff support, and other important operations which occur in hospice.

Hospice aides have additional special training in bereavement and death and dying issues.

STAGES OF GRIEF

Dr. Elisabeth Kubler-Ross was an expert on death and dying issues. She identified five "stages" of grief[1]. It is important to note that all patients have their own unique responses. The aide and other care-givers must support the patient and family through each stage of the dying process. Keep in mind that the stages do not always occur in this order or may appear to occur together. The stages and supportive responses are:

1. **Denial** - This stage occurs usually after the initial diagnosis and the patient responds with shock and denial due to the awareness and knowledge of the fatal or terminal illness.
    Intervention/Care - Patience and willingness to talk are important at this stage.

2. **Anger** - This stage usually follows denial. Patients are appropriately angry and ask "why me?" at this stage as well as during various stages throughout the process.
    Intervention/Care - Treat the patient with understanding and respect, do not return the anger.

3. **Bargaining** - Bargaining occurs when the patient attempts to postpone the illness and death.
    Intervention/Care - If the "bargain" is revealed, listen.

4. **Depression** - Depression is a part of the dying and grieving process. Patients have many things to grieve over, including hair loss, loss of strength and their prior activity level, loss of health, anticipating future

losses, and many others, as unique as the patient and the kind of health problem.

Intervention/Care - Allow the patient to express him/herself fully.

5. Acceptance - Acceptance is the final stage of dying. In this stage, the patient is no longer angry or depressed but has accepted that death is inevitable. Some patients reach a peaceful plateau at this stage.

Intervention/Care - There is no need to encourage talking or activity, simply being with the patient is enough.

[1] Kubler-Ross, E: *On Death and Dying,*
New York, Scribner Publishing Co., 1997.

MATERNAL/NEWBORN CARE

1) Maternal/Newborn Care: Many new mothers and their infants are returning home after shortened inpatient hospital stays. In some programs, new mothers and infants go home 12 to 24 hours after an uncomplicated birth. Some patients are referred to home health care for specific services.

2) General Information: The role of the HHA in these "Home Care Maternity" or "Early Discharge Maternity" programs is very important. There are two patients in the household - the mother and child. Oftentimes there are others, small children who are the siblings of the newborn. Usually the mother cares for the infant, and the HHA provides personal care and a break for the mother.

3) Home Health Aide Goals of Care:
- Patients clean and comfortable and afforded needed rest periods
- Safe assistance with activities of daily living
- Infection control measures maintained
- Other goals

4) Personal Care Considerations: You may be asked to assist the mother with showering. This is particularly true if the mother is uncomfortable due to hemorrhoids or breast milk fullness. Ask the nurse about any questions you may have.

The HHA may also watch the newborn and any other children while the mother takes a shower without being disturbed. Should you care for the infant, document any bowel movements or wet diapers. Meal preparation, snacks for the children, and general assistance, depending on the patient needs and your program, may be required. As always, check your aide assignment sheet or ask the nurse for any questions.

As for all patients and care, explain what you are going to do and what you are doing as you do it.

5) Safety Considerations: It is important to use proper handwashing techniques, especially as infants should be protected against infection.

Although the mother generally is the patient, you may be watching the other children while she is napping or showering. Child care safety considerations must be addressed. Watch that the children are safe in the home environment. Never leave children unattended. Keep small objects, medications, cleaning agents, and plants out of reach of toddlers and small children. If you notice unprotected electrical outlets or other safety concerns, let the nurse know as she/he may address "childhood safety" with the new mother.

Watch for water safety, like pools, bathtubs, buckets of water, etc., which could be hazardous to infants or small children.

6) Documentation Tips: Document the care you provide on the correct form. Some programs have special forms for the "Maternity Patient Programs".

Remember, if the nurse orders a service on the care plan and there is no spot on the aide checklist for that task, write it in longhand on the form under "other".

Document any coordination of care activities.

7) Special Considerations:

____

____

____

NUTRITION CARE

1) Nutrition Care: Nutrition is the nourishment taken in for the body. Nutrition is a process that is comprised of a few parts: the food, drink or other nourishment is consumed; the food is broken down into fuel and absorbed by the body. More and more, good nutrition choices are seen as key to good health!

2) General Information: Home health aides have important roles to play related to nutrition. For examples, the aide care plan, that your supervisor completes, might list the following duties related to nutrition: the kind of diet the patient may be on (for example, for a patient with diabetes, a diabetes diet), any kinds of supplements the patient may be taking (such as Ensure or others), and any fluid or other restrictions (this is particularly true for either cardiac or patients with renal (kidney) failure). In addition, the aide may be asked to prepare meals, know what foods the patient is allergic to or otherwise can not have, shop for food for the homebound patient, assist with feeding and other duties. All of these are important nutrition-related activities that may make the difference between a patient getting stronger and walking or not and a wound healing or not —so the aide plays a very important role!

3) Home Health Aide Goals of Care:
- Optimal nutrition and hydration
- Nutritional and dietary guidelines supported
- Attractive meals prepared and served
- Safe assistance with meal preparation and serving/feeding
- Other goals

4) Personal Care Considerations: The aide care plan may list that the aide should "prepare breakfast". Though unfortunate, your patient may be uncomfortable telling you they have no money with which to purchase food –so they may say they are "not hungry" or "already ate". Remember that it is very important that the patient eat –particularly if the patient has diabetes and your task is to prepare and serve that first meal -breakfast. The nurse may check the refrigerator or the patient's cupboards to check for food in the house. Effective nutrition provides the body with the fuel needed for health, healing, growth and maintenance. Because we must have food for these reasons, notify your supervisor if your patient does not eat or has no food. Some patients receive "Meals on Wheels" or other services. However, it is important that the aide check that the patient is actually eating the delivered food. The nurse can then decide if a nutritionist or a dietitian should be called in to see the patient. These specialists are experts about nutrition. They may be appropriate to be called in for older adult patients with the following health problems: Food allergies and sensitivities, AIDS/HIV and wasting syndrome, drug/nutrient/food interactions, cancer, diabetes mellitus, digestive disorders (including patients who receive "tube" feedings), cardiac (heart) patients as they may have a salt and fat restricted diet, patients needing weight loss for health, those with osteoporosis, wounds, and others. Ask your nursing supervisor –she may help the patient by calling in the dietitian or nutritionist.

5) Safety Considerations: According to the U.S. Government, a growing body of research shows that fruits and vegetables are critical to promoting and maintaining good health. They contain essential vitamins, minerals, and fiber that may help prevent chronic diseases. If you are food shopping for a patient (or for yourself and your family) to get a healthy variety, think about colors! Try to get a wide range of colors in fruits and vegetables. Also a wide range of nutrients can be found in grains, vegetables, fruits, milk and dairy and meats and beans. The government has a web site located at www.MyPyramid.gov that contains the latest news, information and resources about food and nutrition.

If you have a patient who has trouble swallowing — never force any kind of food or fluid. Call your supervisor for any questions. Similarly, if you have a patient who is very ill, such as those with end-stage disease or cancer, they may not wish to eat or drink and this is a normal part of the dying process –ask the dietitian or your nursing supervisor for any questions.

6) Documentation Tips: Document/check off the tasks you completed as specified on the aide care plan.

Document if the patient refuses food (and fluids, etc.) and why, if known.

Document the patient intake.

Document the patient weights and report to the nursing supervisor if the weight is above or below any level set by the supervisor (e.g., a weight gain in a cardiac patient can be a sign that they are gaining fluid and may be getting sicker) and the nurse would need to know this right away.

Remember, if the nurse orders a service on the care plan and there is no place on the checklist for that specific task; write it in longhand on the aide care plan form under "other".

7) Special Considerations: A nutritious, balanced diet with a variety of foods is needed for optimal health. Many home health care patients are very sick, frail, or healing from surgery. It is an important aspect of our work that we encourage these patients to eat, when they are able to do so.

OLDER ADULT CARE

1) Older Adult Care: Many of the patients we care for in home care are older adults. There are physiological changes associated with aging which are a normal part of the aging process.

Please refer to "Constipation Care", "Arthritis Care" or other specific patient problems for a more in-depth discussion of these possible patient care needs.

2) General Information: Things to consider when caring for older adults or elders are that their senses generally diminish or become less acute with age. This can mean patients are "hard of hearing" or deaf and/or have vision problems and need glasses. Their ability to smell and to taste food may also decrease, foods and spices may no longer "taste the same". In addition, bones lose density, which can cause osteoporosis. This can contribute to brittle bones which can fracture, or break easily, with a fall or pressure. Skin can become tissue paper thin, tear, break down (pressure ulcers), or bruise easily. For all of these reasons, a nutritious diet and a safe home environment are important components of supporting and maintaining the patient's independence at home.

Some older adult patients may be set in their beliefs and values. Respect their decisions to do things in their own ways unless not appropriate or unsafe.

3) Home Health Aide Goals of Care:
- Patient clean, safe and comfortable
- Infection control measures maintained
- Medication compliance
- Adequate hydration and nutrition
- Patient area clean and tidy
- Bowel protocol monitored and maintained

- Energy and joint conservation
- Safe assistance with activities of daily living
- Patient safely assisted with home exercise program (as shown by therapist or nurse supervisor)
- Personal emergency response system (PERS) nearby
- Other goals

4) Personal Care Considerations: Skin care is very important for older adults, particularly if they are bedridden or sit in one position for lengthy periods. These situations may cause skin breakdown. Nutritional deficiencies, some medications, and illness can all contribute to the risk of your patient's skin breaking down and forming pressure ulcers.

Many older adult patients have arthritis so in the mornings it may be more painful to move joints during bathing. Let the patient tell you how to move them. When bathing your patient, inspect the patient's skin for any breakdown, redness, or changes from your last visit. Be very gentle when turning these patients as some patients have "tissue paper" like skin that is very fragile and tears easily. If there is a skin tear, place a bandage over the area to prevent further injury. Report this to the nurse who may check for oozing or infection. Use a pull sheet to gently reposition the patient if necessary. Because the skin is so fragile and tears easily, notify the nurse if you notice any skin changes.

Communications are very important, particularly with a confused patient or hearing impaired patient. Some patients like to talk about "old times" and reminisce about the past. Listen attentively and respect your patient by not talking "baby talk" or raising your voice. It is often more helpful to rephrase what you are saying if your patient is hard of hearing or speak more slowly and clearly rather than speaking louder. Assist your patient with caring for hearing aids and keeping glasses clean.

As for all patients and care, explain what you are going to do and what you are doing as you do it.

5) Safety Considerations: Older adult patients may have poor balance or slow reflexes and are more at risk for fractures and other injuries with falls. In addition, multiple medications may increase the chance for falls. Falls can be avoided by clearing the patient area and household walkways from clutter where possible. Be sure to leave assistive/adaptive devices (walker, quad cane) and the phone within the patient's reach for use and safety. Notify the supervisor if the walker, cane, or other equipment appears unsafe.

Some elders who live alone, or are alone during the day, have a personal emergency response system or PERS, in case they need help. If your patients have one, encourage them to wear their button as required for this technology to work.

Before leaving your patient's home, place the phone near the patient for safety or be sure the phone is left within the patient's reach. Remind patient of safe behaviors (e.g. no climbing to reach something, use their assistive device all the time, etc).

6) Documentation Tips: Document the care you provided on the aide documentation form.

If your patient tells you they fell since your last visit, always report this and document according to agency policy.

Document the date and amount of bowel movement as some patients have difficulty moving their bowels or are constipated. Notify the nurse if there is any bleeding with bowel movements or if the patient has not had one in _____ days (ask the nurse to specify how frequently a bowel movement should occur and when the nurse should be contacted).

Document any observed changes in skin, appetite, alertness, orientation, falls, etc. Also document any co-ordination of care activities. Remember, if the nurse orders a service on the care plan and there is no spot on the aide checklist for that task, write it in longhand on the form under "other".

Document any coordination of care activities.

7) **Special Considerations:** Older adults can get dehydrated very easily from not drinking enough fluids, taking certain medications, extreme heat and other reasons. Dehydration as well as infection can cause confusion in the patient, in addition to other health problems. Check with the nurse, and if approved, offer the patient fluids throughout your visit. This is important to check with the nurse about because some patients have heart or kidney problems and their fluid intake may be restricted

____

____

____

1) Colostomy/Ileostomy/Urostomy Care: A colostomy is a surgical creation of an artificial opening of the colon through the abdominal wall. Colostomies can be temporary or permanent and can have a single opening or two openings, called a double-barreled colostomy. The part of the colon that protrudes above the skin level is the stoma (hence the term "colostomy") and provides the outlet for intestinal waste. Sometimes colostomies are permanent, though some are temporary.

A colostomy is performed for various reasons, including cancer, obstructions in the bowel, and severe abdominal wounds. Colostomies also affect young individuals who have diseases like irritable bowel syndrome or Crohn's disease as well as older adults with cancer or obstructions. An ileostomy is a surgically created opening in the abdominal wall through which digested food passes.

A urostomy is a surgical creation or diversion of the urine flow to be collected in an appliance worn on the abdomen. The urine flows into the pouch which can be emptied into a container or into the toilet.

Please refer to "Cancer Care" or other specific patient problems for a more in depth discussion of these possible patient care needs.

2) General Information: A colostomy, ileostomy or urostomy is a traumatic experience for any patient. It affects their daily activities and is a loss of the "normal way" to have a bowel movement. It is a significant change in body self-image. Patients with colostomies have body image issues to address. The adjustment period, the months after the colostomy, can be the most difficult. Many patients live long, healthy lives and adapt well to living with a colostomy. In fact, patients can participate in sports and other activities as they did prior to surgery.

As with the colostomy or ileostomy, the urostomy is a different way for urine to leave the body and can be emotionally upsetting to the patient. This is a loss, just like losing any other "regular" body function or part. The urostomy is permanent, but once healing occurs the patient may resume all previous activity.

3) Home Health Aide Goals of Care:
- Patient clean, safe and comfortable
- Safe assistance with activities of daily living
- Minimized skin problems through care
- Infection control measures maintained
- Privacy and dignity provided during care
- Other goals

4) Personal Care Considerations: Some patients will not want to see their colostomy. This is their choice and should be respected while you are providing personal care.

Skin irritation or other changes from drainage may cause skin breakdown and must be reported to the nurse. Urine and stool are very irritating to the skin and leakage under the appliance must be reported immediately to the patient, family, or nurse, depending upon who is learning the care.

Keep in mind, if your patients are also receiving chemotherapy or radiation therapy and had their ostomy because of cancer, they may be tired and need rest periods between care activities.

As for all patients and care, explain what you are going to do and what you are doing as you do it. You may also be asked to assist with emptying the colostomy/urostomy bag. Ask your nurse for specific instructions. If you have any questions, always ask your supervisor first!

5) Safety Considerations: When providing care, gently care for the skin around the stoma as it is a new surgical opening.

Be careful not to drip soap on the stoma or the surrounding skin as this can cause severe irritation.

Ask the patient's nurse for questions you may have. The nurse will be providing the actual hands-on care to the new stoma colostomy site. Sometimes when patients have long-term colostomies, they should be caring for the ostomy site themselves. In those instances where the patients cannot provide their own care, the nurse will direct you. Teaching of the care is provided by the nurse. **If urine is not flowing into the urostomy bag, this should be immediately reported to the nurse.**

6) Documentation Tips: If your patient does not have a bowel movement for two days, this should be documented and reported to the nurse.

Skin irritation should be reported to the nurse right away.

Write the care you provided on the aide form.

Remember, if the nurse orders a specific task on the assignment sheet, it should be checked off on your documentation form.

Be sure to sign your name clearly, the patient's name, your title, and the date and time of the care you provided.

Remember, if the nurse orders a service on the care plan and there is no spot on the aide checklist for that task, write it in longhand on the form under "other".

Document any coordination of care activities.

7) **Special Considerations:** Effective nutrition and dietary habits are very important to the comfort and well-being of the patient with a colostomy. A nutritionist or dietitian may be involved in your patient's care.

An enterostomal or wound nurse (called a wound ostomy continence nurse, or WOCN) may also be involved in the care of these patients.

The patient may have been sent home with a list of foods to avoid because they may cause pain and gas. These foods can include: milk, spicy foods, beans, cabbage, carbonated drinks, onions, beer, and cucumbers. Fruits and fruit juice may cause frequent bowel movements or diarrhea. Foods which can cause increased odor are onions, eggs, fish, and broccoli. Generally, items/foods that caused gas prior to surgery will still cause gas. Try to prepare foods that are on the "okay list". Ask your supervisor about foods which may be okay and those that may be questionable.

Odors may be offensive to the patient. There are products available to alleviate this problem. Ask the nurse for direction and be sure to report to the nurse if the patient seems to be low on supplies.

PAIN MANAGEMENT CARE

1) Pain Management Care: It is important to remember that patients are the experts on how they feel – especially about their pain. Pain is a subjective feeling (how it feels to a specific patient) and is an individual response to the cause.

2) General Information: There are many different ways your patients will communicate to you about their pain. A common way to rate pain is a pain scale, usually measured from 0 to 10 with 0 being no pain and 10 being the worst pain. They can also describe pain in different ways, such as a dull ache, throbbing, or "sensitive to the touch". Some patients won't say anything at all, but may be tearful, pacing, restless, anxious, nauseated or have numerous other manifestations of pain.

When you believe your patient is experiencing pain, or has a change in pain status, such as a new or increased pain, contact the nurse.

Many pain medications can cause constipation. It is important for the aide to help patients keep track of their bowel movements and urination. If your patient is constipated, report this to the nurse who will start the patient on a bowel regimen.

3) Home Health Aide Goals of Care:
- Patient clean, safe and comfortable
- Pain managed effectively per patient report
- Infection control measures maintained
- Patient area clean and tidy
- Safe assistance with activities of daily living
- Medication compliance
- Observes and reports pain increase to nurse
- Bowel protocol monitored and maintained for patient comfort
- Other goals

4) Personal Care Considerations: If your patients are uncomfortable, they may not be able to concentrate on the bath or other personal care that you are there to provide. Ask patients what will make them more comfortable. Sometimes a soothing backrub or hand or foot massage can assist your patients in becoming more comfortable. Relaxation or diversional techniques may be helpful. Offer to play their favorite music, or other activities that they enjoy.

Sometimes patients sleep in and may have "slept past" their pain medication time. In these cases, it is important to tell the patient what time it is. Call the nurse and ask about staying there with the patient, while the medication is taken, and allowing it time to work, before proceeding with care (This usually takes about 15-20 minutes).

Remember, the patient's pain is real to him or her. Work with the other team members to increase comfort and resolve the pain.

As for all patients and care, explain what you are going to do and what you are doing as you do it.

5) Safety Considerations: Sometimes patients with pain or on pain medications become restless. Try to clear a pathway between patient areas, so that the patient doesn't slip and fall.

Some pain medications may cause patients to be sleepy or drowsy. Allow enough time for the patient to wake up and not be groggy, particularly if you want the patient to walk or stand. Support the patient with either of these activities for safety.

Generally, for patients on pain medications, allow them time to sit on the side of the bed before moving to a standing position. This "dangling" can help with the dizziness that some patients experience.

The patient may use ice or heat for pain relief. Remind the patient to protect the skin where the ice or heat will be applied. Cover ice bags with a towel or check heat setting for safety.

6) Documentation Tips: Document the care you provided on the aide form.

Document the patient's complaints related to pain and your call to the office, if you called.

Note what the patient's usual pain is on a scale of 0 to 10 when the patient is asked.

Remember, if the nurse orders a service on the care plan and there is no spot on the aide checklist for that task, write it in longhand on the form under "other".

Document any coordination of care activities.

7) Special Considerations: Signs of pain include: grimacing, furrowed brow, perspiring, increased breath sounds or sighs and changes in pulse and restlessness levels. Responses to pain and signs of pain vary widely and your patient can look "okay" and still report pain. Your patient is the expert on his or her pain. Pain identification tools are being used more extensively, happy faces and/or the number scale. Your agency will review this information with you.

____

____

____

PNEUMONIA CARE

1) Pneumonia Care: Pneumonia is a serious lung infection. Elders can be particularly at risk, such as when having the "flu". During the "flu season", health professionals recommend that older adults get the flu shot. Unfortunately, there are many strains of flu and the shot is usually for a particular strain.

2) General Information: Patients, particularly older patients, are often admitted to home care after being hospitalized with pneumonia. In the hospital they received strong antibiotics to kill the infection, and fluids to loosen the congestion and prevent them from being dehydrated. Sometimes patients are cared for at home after being seen at the doctor's office and started on antibiotic treatment. Either way, this important care is continued. Generally, patients recovering from pneumonia will tire easily at first, but slowly return to their normal activities.

3) Home Health Aide Goals of Care:
- Patient clean, safe and comfortable
- Patient area clean and tidy
- Safe assistance with and increase in activities of daily living
- Infection control measures maintained
- Nutritious meals and fluids of patient's choice prepared and served
- Bowel protocol monitored and maintained
- Emotional support
- Energy conservation
- Other goals

4) Personal Care Considerations: After hospitalization, many older adults lose some of their mobility and strength. A physical or occupational therapist or the nurse may show you range of motion exercises for your patient. As always, only provide the services listed on your assignment sheet, or as designated by the nurse or therapist. Call your supervisor if you are unclear or have questions.

If your assignment is to prepare meals, ask patients what they prefer. Try to serve nutritious foods for your patients and sit with them while they eat. Offer fluids of choice and encourage liquids if your patient is not on fluid restrictions.

After pneumonia, patients are usually sent home and encouraged to cough and deep breathe to improve their lung capacity. Ask the nurse for instructions about this. Your patient may be also taking medications through an inhaler.

As for all patients and care, explain what you are going to do and what you are doing as you do it.

5) Safety Considerations: Pneumonia is a very serious infection. If you take the patient's temperature or respiratory rate and it is higher than usual or not normal, call the nurse. In addition, call the nurse if the patient's coughing does not decrease or improve over time.

Fall safety: The patient may be very weak. Give the patient time to adjust to sitting on the side of the bed before attempting to stand or walk.

If your patient has increased phlegm or congestion or a change in color, is coughing more, can't catch his or her breath or feels shorter of breath, can't talk due to shortness of breath or coughing, becomes confused, or has other, new, or different symptoms, call the nurse and report these changes/symptoms.

The patient may require instruction to properly dispose of tissues used to collect coughed-up mucous. For infection control purposes, it is important to be sure that tissues and a bag for their disposal are available both when you are present and after you leave.

If you notice that patients are not taking their antibiotics or other medications, call the nurse.

6) Documentation Tips: Document the care you provided on the aide documentation form.

Document the patient's bowel movements and intake and output on the form.

Document the patient's vital signs on the form and/or the calendar that remains in the patient's home, based on your organization's policies.

Remember, if the nurse orders a service on the care plan and there is no spot on the aide checklist for that task, write it in longhand on the form under "other".

Document any coordination of care activities.

7) Special Considerations: Always wear gloves when assisting patients with excessive mucous to prevent transferring germs to yourself and others.

____

____

____

POST SURGICAL CARE (CARE OF THE PATIENT AFTER SURGERY)

1) **Post Surgical Care:** Post-surgical or postoperative care is the care that occurs after patients have had surgery and are continuing care and recuperating in their own home. Readers may also refer to "Bone/Fracture/Joint Replacement Care" or "Pain Management Care" guidelines.

2) **General Information:** Surgery care can include patients who have had their appendix out, a heart procedure such as a bypass graft or a pacemaker, a colostomy, or many others. Some patients may come home with "tubes" attached to drainage bags. All patients after surgery can be prone to certain kinds of problems or infections. The aide plays an important role in noticing any changes in patients and reporting these to the nurse. The aide also provides needed personal care and activities of daily living assistance to these patients.

3) **Home Health Aide Goals of Care:**
- Patient clean, safe and comfortable
- Pain managed effectively per patient report
- Patient comfort and safety
- Patient area clean and tidy
- Safe assistance with activities of daily living
- Patient assisted with and has increased mobility
- Infection control measures maintained
- Nutritious meals prepared and served
- Observation and reporting of pain or discomfort
- Emotional support
- Bowel protocol monitored and maintained
- Other goals

4) Personal Care Considerations: Generally, the surgical site may be covered by a dressing when the patient first comes home from the hospital. **The nurse cares for the wound. However, if the HHA notices drainage through the dressing, bleeding, or any other changes or problems, they must be reported to the nurse immediately.** If necessary, remind the patient to take the pain medication prior to bathing, ambulation, and other activity.

The patient may feel a pulling or discomfort at the site for some time. It is important that the sutures, stitches, or staples remain clean, dry, and intact. Patients know when and how to move, because their discomfort guides them. Do not hurry the patient who has a surgical wound, as this may injure the patient and disrupt the healing process. Patients who stay in bed for too long may need to be gently encouraged to move about to prevent complications, such as pneumonia, urinary tract infection, or possible blood clots. Always ask the nurse any questions you may have about the patient's activity level.

Do not get the dressing wet as this may contribute to an infection. Provide your personal care everywhere but around the surgical site. Should the wound get wet, such as by a spill, call the nurse; the dressing will need to be changed by the nurse.

The therapist or nurse may teach you exercises to perform with the patient. Provide these exercises as shown, and only as directed by the nurse or therapist.

As for all patients and care, explain what you are going to do and what you are doing as you do it.

5) Safety Considerations: Support your patient, as necessary when standing or walking. Encourage the use of assistive devices, like a walker or quad cane, as shown by the nurse or therapist.

Sometimes when patients cough, they have pain. Using a pillow to "splint" or protect the incision helps lessen the pain after coughing. Be careful with "tubes" that are in patients. Care should be taken not to have tension on the tubing or let the containers hang from the site. These tubes should not be dislodged. The nurse can show you how to attach them properly. If there is any problem with the patient's tube, call the nurse.

If you notice changes in the patient such as increased or changed pain, fever, or if the patient complains of urinary burning, chest pain, pain when walking, or other complaints or symptoms, call the nurse.

6) Documentation Tips: Document the care provided on the aide form.

Document bowel movements, temperature, other vital signs, urinary output on the form, as per your organization's policies.

Remember, if the nurse orders a service on the care plan and there is no spot on the aide checklist for that task, write it in longhand on the form under "other".

Document any coordination of care activities.

7) Special Considerations: Always follow standard precautions while providing care.

____

____

____

PRESSURE ULCER CARE

1) Pressure Ulcer Care: A pressure ulcer is an inflammation, sore, or opening in the skin, usually over a bony prominence. Formerly pressure ulcers were called decubitus ulcers. Pressure ulcers result from prolonged pressure on the skin to the affected area. There is an old saying which is very true: "The best treatment for bedsores is prevention".

According to the Agency for Healthcare Research and Quality (AHRQ), a pressure ulcer is an injury usually caused by unrelieved pressure that damages the skin and underlying tissue. Pressure ulcers are also called bedsores and range in severity from mild (minor skin reddening) to severe (deep craters down to muscle and bone). Pressure ulcers are staged (or categorized) in four stages. They range from Stage I to Stage IV on their severity. For more information, see the website www.wocn.org.

Unrelieved pressure on the skin squeezes tiny blood vessels, which supply the skin with nutrients and oxygen. When the skin is starved of nutrients and oxygen for too long, the tissue dies and a pressure ulcer forms. Skin reddening that disappears after pressure is removed is normal and not a pressure ulcer.

Other factors cause pressure ulcers too. If a person slides down in the bed or chair, blood vessels can stretch or bend and cause pressure ulcers. Moisture from incontinence or perspiration may also contribute to the development of pressure ulcers. Even slight rubbing or friction on the skin may cause minor pressure ulcers. These injuries happen to anyone who stays in one position too long, even if they are able to walk, but often these patients are paralyzed on one side, in their upper body, or in their lower body.

TISSUE UNDER PRESSURE
Body Weight

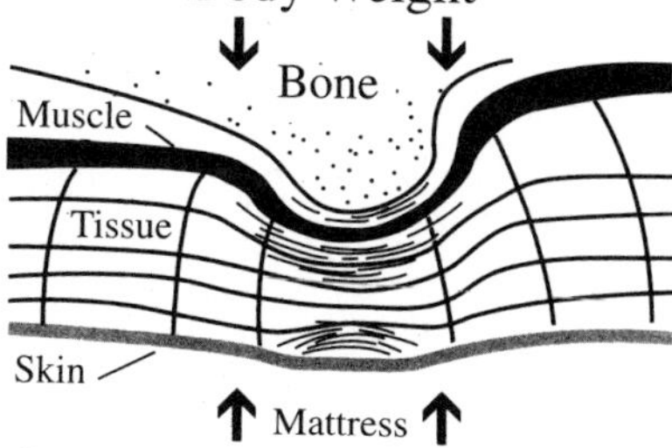

2) General Information: The aide plays a key role in the prevention of skin breakdown and pressure ulcer formation. Patients who lie in bed or sit for extended periods of time in one position are at risk for skin breakdown. This means that you must change or help the patient to change their position to allow the skin to breathe and receive needed blood and oxygen, which is cut off when the patient remains in one position.

3) Home Health Aide Goals of Care:

- Patient clean, safe and comfortable
- Skin intact and personal care provided
- Effective nutrition and hydration maintained
- Infection control measures maintained
- Joints maintained in functional position
- Bowel protocol monitored and maintained
- Other goals

4) Personal Care Considerations: When bathing your patient, observe the patient's skin for sign of breakdown. This includes all bony areas, such as the coccyx (tail bone), the hip bones, shoulder blades, and others.

Turn your patient frequently, at least every two hours. Use antipressure supplies that are available, such as heel protectors, dense foam or other special mattresses, cushions for the wheelchair and many others.

If you identify that the patient needs pressure ulcer care or prevention supplies, contact the nurse. The nurse will speak with the physician to obtain the order for needed skin protection supplies.

It is very important to check for and change soiled clothes and liners on incontinent patients frequently as urine is an acid and can contribute to skin breakdown.

As for all patients and care, explain what you are going to do and what you are doing as you do it.

5) Safety Considerations: Turn or reposition your patient at intervals as determined by the assignment sheet or the nurse. You may also have the family watch you so they can turn the patient when you are not there.

If you identify ANY skin change or potential problems, speak to the nurse. Pressure ulcers can become infected and cause other serious infections.

The patient may benefit from special pillows or mattresses that assist in preventing skin breakdown.

6) Documentation Tips: Document the services you provided on the aide form.

If you identify changes in the skin, note these on your form, and follow-up with a call to the nurse.

Remember, if the nurse orders a service on the care plan and there is no spot on the aide checklist for that task, write it in longhand on the form under "other".

7) Special Considerations: Effective nutrition, hydration, position changes, and home exercise can assist in the prevention of skin breakdown. Try to have the patient stay off the open or affected area. Some patients have very poor appetites or even refuse to eat. Healing in these or other instances can sometimes seem impossible. The goal then becomes keeping the patient comfortable and the wound/ulcer clean and infection free. Talk to the nurse if your patient's wound is not progressing or healing. Encourage your patient to eat vegetables, fruit, and proteins. The nurse may contact the doctor for a dietitian or a nutritionist to visit the patient.

Offer juices and/or nutritional supplements if ordered on your assignment sheet as well as protein supplements while in home if it is part of the care plan.

____

____

____

TUBERCULOSIS (TB) CARE

1) Tuberculosis Care: Tuberculosis (TB) is an infection that generally presents symptoms in the respiratory system, although it also can be found in the kidneys and spinal column. Tuberculosis is generally transmitted by the inhalation or ingestion of infected air droplets. There is an increase in the number of patients with tuberculosis all over the world. Patients whose immune systems are weakened from AIDS or chemotherapy treatments for cancer are particularly susceptible.

2) General Information: Tuberculosis is a respiratory disease that spreads through the air when untreated. The bacteria can "hide" for long periods which is why health care workers are tested at regular intervals for exposure. Your patient with TB may be on multiple medications. It is vital for patients to regularly take and finish these medications. Treatment lasts up to one year or even longer. Patients with TB are usually hospitalized for the beginning of the long-term medication treatment. This inpatient stay also assists in limiting the spread of the infection, because the patient starts immediately on the medication therapy. The inpatient stay also provides an opportunity to educate patients about this disease.

3) Home Health Aide Goals of Care:
- Patient clean, safe and comfortable
- Patient area clean and tidy
- Infection control measures maintained
- Medication compliance maintained/monitored
- Safe assistance with activities of daily living
- Optimal hydration and nutrition maintained
- Other goals

4) Personal Care Considerations: Patients with tuberculosis can tire easily or become short of breath and may need rest periods between tasks. Fevers and sweating may require the bed linens to be changed more often. The occupational therapist may assist with energy conservation measures.

Taking vital signs and weights are very important for patients with TB. Ask the nurse for any special instructions.

As for all patients and care, explain what you are going to do and what you are doing as you do it.

5) Safety Considerations: Adhere to standard precautions and check with your supervisor for the need for specific protective equipment related to TB. You may be fitted for a special mask in some cases.

Used tissues with mucous must be disposed of carefully. Adhere to your organization's infection control guidelines. Provide easy access to tissues and a paper bag or wastebasket to dispose of used tissues.

Should patients mention they are not taking any or all of their medications, report this to the nurse.

6) Documentation Tips: Document the care you provided to the patient.

Document what you observe during the visit.

Remember, if the nurse orders a service on the care plan and there is no spot on the aide checklist for that task, write it in longhand on the form under "other".

Document any coordination of care activities.

7) Special Considerations:

____

____

____

URINARY CATHETER/CONDOM CATHETER/SUPRAPUBIC TUBE CARE

1) Urinary Catheter/Condom Catheter/Suprapubic Tube Care: Many patients are referred to home care with an indwelling catheter. An indwelling or foley type catheter is a sterile tube which is inserted into the bladder. Common reasons that patients have catheters include bladder "atony" (a loss of muscle), incontinence, residual urine problems (when patients do not empty their bladder, sometimes causing infection), and others. Other patients may use "condom" catheters which are external urinary collection devices. The aide may also assist in this care (e.g. putting the condom catheter on the patient).

Some patients have a tube inserted surgically directly into the bladder. This is called a suprapubic tube (supra means above and pubic refers to the pubic bone). The catheter enters the body low on the abdomen. This tube is connected to a leg or constant drainage bag just like a urinary catheter.

2) General Information: Patients with catheters may be bedridden or bedbound with a stroke (CVA) or other medical problems.

Patients with a suprapubic tube may have neurological or mobility problems preventing use of the toilet.

3) Home Health Aide Goals of Care:
- Patient clean, safe and comfortable
- Urinary catheter care safely provided
- Infection control measures maintained
- Bowel protocol monitored and maintained
- Minimized skin problems through personal care
- Safe assistance with activities of daily living
- Excellent peri-care
- Other goals

4) Personal Care Considerations: When providing personal care and catheter care, you are in a good position to identify problems with the patient's catheter. Any problems noted or identified should be referred to your supervisor.

Sometimes patients use a leg bag during the day to contain urine.

Problems to be noted and discussed with your nurse supervisor include: blood in the urine, fever or chills, constipation (constipation can put pressure on the patient's bladder), patient complaints of pain, burning, or bladder spasms, the catheter falling "out", increased sediment or particles in the urine bag, leaking from around the catheter, bleeding, or other problems or changes.

Perfumes, powders or lotions should not be applied around the catheter. During the bath, soap and water should be used to clean around the urinary opening and to gently wash.

As for all patients and care, explain what you are going to do and what you are doing as you do it.

5) Safety Considerations: The urinary drainage bag or leg bag should always be lower than the patient's bladder – but never on the floor. Remember that the floor is very dirty and hygiene is very important in preventing urinary as well as other infections. Always wash your hands and use gloves before and after providing any care with the patient's catheter or catheter bag.

Should the suprapubic tube fall out, time is very important. A new tube must be reinserted by the nurse within a few hours. Call the nurse as soon as this happens!

The catheter and drainage tubing should only be separated when changing bags, and this should be done by the aide only after being shown and directed to do this by the nurse. When changing drainage bags, wipe the tip of the bag tubing with an alcohol swab before inserting into the catheter opening. For any questions, call the nurse supervisor. The catheter should be secured, not just hanging down, as this can dislodge the catheter or cause discomfort. If the tubing gets kinked, or bent, the urine cannot drain down, and this can contribute to infections. The collection bag should be maintained below the level of the bladder at all times. Ask your nurse about your organization's policy about securing urinary catheters and the safe use/application of leg straps.

6) Documentation Tips: Write the care you provided on the aide form.

Document the specific urine output from the catheter, in millimeters, if specified on the plan.
Your organization may also teach you how to measure the urine and to clean the drainage bag. The method and the frequency of this cleaning will be directed by the nurse.

Remember, if the nurse orders a service on the care plan and there is no spot on the aide checklist for that task, write it in longhand on the form under "other".

Document any coordination of care activities.

7) Special Considerations: Because nutrition and hydration are important to the maintenance of the bladder and other body systems, adhere to the aide assignment sheet related to offering fluids or dietary supplements as ordered and directed by the nurse. Ask your patients which juices or fluids they prefer, such as cranberry juice. Offer these fluids of choice often, as approved by the nurse.

WOUND CARE

1) Wound Care: Wound care is a common reason for patients to be admitted to home care. A wound is any injury or opening to the skin.

Please refer to "Pressure Ulcer Care", "Pain Management Care", and "Postsurgical Care" or other specific patient problems for a more in-depth discussion of these possible patient care needs

2) General Information: The kinds of wound problems cared for in home care include: pressure ulcers, dermal wounds, ostomy wound sites, postoperative surgical sites, and others. The nurse is very involved and provides the actual care, teaching and training, and on-going assessment of the wound and the patient. The aide has an important role in observation and reporting any change in the wound.

3) Home Health Aide Goals of Care:
- Patient clean, safe and comfortable
- Patient area clean and tidy
- Normal blood sugar (for patient)
- Safe assistance with activities of daily living
- Infection control measures maintained
- Adequate/optimal patient protein intake
- Observes and reports any changes in drainage, the dressing, etc.
- Patient assisted with and has increased mobility
- Other goals

4) Personal Care Considerations: The role of the aide is very important in wound care. Duties such as vital signs, including taking/checking the patient's temperature, talking to the patient about "how they are doing" during their bath, and inspecting their skin, can all contribute to improving patient care.

The aide usually does not provide wound care, but cares for patient's personal care needs and assists in completing activities of daily living. You may be asked to "reinforce" a leaky dressing by applying gauze to it until the nurse arrives.

Prepare and serve nutritious meals to the patient, if that is a part of your assignment. Nutrition and hydration (fluids) play an important role in wound healing.

As for all patients and care, explain what you are going to do and what you are doing as you do it.

5) Safety Considerations: As with all patients, maintain standard precautions. Use effective handwashing techniques when providing care to your patients. Note any drainage or change in the amount of drainage and report this to the nurse. Also, if the patient has increased pain, report this to the nurse and note this in your documentation. If drainage becomes visible through the dressing, call the nurse.

6) Documentation Tips: Document the care you have provided on the aide form.

Remember, if the nurse orders a service on the care plan and there is no spot on the aide checklist for that task, write it in longhand on the form under "other".

Document any coordination of care activities.

7) Special Considerations: If possible, and if there are no restrictions, the patient may need a high protein diet for healing. Ask the nurse or dietitian for instructions.

____

____

____

PART THREE

APPENDIXES

APPENDIX A

HOME CARE AND HOSPICE ABBREVIATIONS

The following abbreviations are those that may be seen in home care and hospice practice. Your organization may also have an approved abbreviation list for documentation in their clinical records. Always ask your supervisor for clarification about any abbreviation that is not clear. In addition, your organization may have a list of "Do Not Use" abbreviations. This is for safety reasons. Whenever possible, spell out terms for clarity and safety in communications.

ABD	Abdomen
AC	Before Meals
AD	Assistive Device
ADLs	Activities of Daily Living
AIDS	Acquired Immune Deficiency Syndrome
AKA	Above Knee Amputation
ALS	Amyotrophic Lateral Sclerosis (Lou Gehrig's Disease)
AM	Morning
AMI	Acute Myocardial Infarction
APHA	American Public Health Association
ASD	Atrial Septal Defect
BKA	Below Knee Amputation
BM	Bowel Movement
BP	Blood Pressure
BPH	Benign Prostatic Hypertrophy
BR	Bathroom
BRP	Bathroom Privileges
BS	Blood Sugar
C	(centigrade) Celsius

$\overline{C}$	With
CA	Cancer
CAD	Coronary Artery Disease
CBC	Complete Blood Count
CDCP	Centers for Disease Control & Prevention
CHAP	Community Health Accreditation Program
CHHA	Certified Home Health Aide
CHPNA	Certified Hospice and Palliative Nursing Assistant
cm	Centimeter
CMS	Centers for Medicare and Medicare Services
COPD	Chronic Obstructive Pulmonary Disease
CoPs	Conditions of Participation
CPAP	Continuous Positive Airway Pressure
CPM	Continuous Passive Motion
CPR	Cardiopulmonary Resuscitation
C & S	Culture and Sensitivity
CVA	Cerebral Vascular Accident
CXR	Chest X Ray
DJD	Degenerative Joint Disease
DM	Diabetes Mellitus
DME	Durable Medical Equipment
DNR	Do Not Resuscitate
DOE	Dyspnea on Exertion
DRG	Diagnosis Related Group
DX	Diagnosis
ECG (EKG)	Electrocardiogram
ED	Emergency Department
ESRD	End Stage Renal Disease
ER	Emergency Room
ET	Enterostomal Therapist
F	Fahrenheit

FBS	Fasting Blood Sugar
FHR	Fetal Heart Rate
FX	Fracture
GI	Gastrointestinal
G-tube (GT)	Gastrostomy Tube
gtts.	Drops
GU	Genitourinary
H2O	Water
HF	Heart Failure
HHA	Home Health Aide or Home Health Agency
HHC	Home Health Care
HIM	Health Insurance Manual
HIPAA	Health Insurance Portability & Accountability Act
HME	Home Medical Equipment
HOB	Head of Bed
HOH	Hard of Hearing
HPNA	Hospice & Palliative Nurse Association
HR	Heart Rate
HS	At Bedtime
HTN	Hypertension
IDDM	Insulin Dependent Diabetes Mellitus
IM	Intramuscular
I & O	Intake and Output
IPPB	Intermittent Positive Pressure Breathing
IV	Intravenous
JCAHO	Joint Commission on Accreditation of Healthcare Organizations
L	Left
LE	Lower Extremity
LLE	Left Lower Extremity
LLL	Left Lower Lobe
LLQ	Left Lower Quadrant
LOC	Level of Consciousness
LPN	Licensed Practical Nurse

LUE	Left Upper Extremity
LUQ	Left Upper Quadrant
LVN	Licensed Vocational Nurse
MI	Myocardial Infarction
MOW	Meals on Wheels
MSS	Medical Social Services
MSW	Medical Social Work
NAHC	National Association for Home Care & Hospice
NG tube	Nasogastric Tube
NHP	Nursing Home Placement
NHPCO	National Hospice & Palliative Care Organization
NIDDM	Non-insulin Dependent Diabetes Mellitus
noc	Night Time
NPDA	National Private Duty Association
NIH	National Institutes of Health
NPO	Nothing By Mouth
NTG	Nitroglycerin
OASIS	Outcome Assessment Information Set
O2	Oxygen
OBQM	Outcome-Based Quality Monitoring
OBS	Organic Brain Syndrome
OD	Right Eye
OOB	Out of Bed
OS	Left Eye
OT	Occupational Therapist
OSHA	Occupational Safety & Health Administration
OT	Occupational Therapy
P	Pulse
P4P	Pay for Performance
PI	Performance Improvement
PCA	Patient-Controlled Analgesia
PERLA	Pupils Equal, React to Light & Accomodation

PICC (line)	Peripherally Inserted Central Catheter
PKU	Phenylketonuria
PM	Afternoon
PO	By Mouth (orally)
POC	Plan of Care
POT	Plan of Treatment
PPE	Personal Protective Equipment
PPS	Prospective Payment System
PRN	As Needed
pt	Patient
PT	Physical Therapy
PVD	Peripheral Vascular Disease
R	Right or Respirations
Rehab	Rehabilitation
RLE	Right Lower Extremity
RLL	Right Lower Lobe
R/O	Rule Out
ROM	Range of Motion
RN	Registered Nurse
RR	Respiratory Rate
RUE	Right Upper Extremity
Rx	Prescription
SL (sl)	Sublingual
S-LP	Speech-Language Pathology
SNV	Skilled Nursing Visit
SOB	Shortness of Breath
S/P	Status Post
SR	Side Rail
SL	Sublingual
S/S	Signs & Symptoms
SSA	Social Security Administration
STAT	Immediately
STD	Sexually Transmitted Diesease
SX	Symptoms
T	Temperature
TB	Tuberculosis

TENS	Transcutaneous Electrical Nerve Stimulation
TIA	Transient Ischemic Attack
THR	Total Hip Replacement
TKR	Total Knee Replacement
TO	Telephone Order
TPN	Total Parenteral Nutrition
TPR	Temperature, Pulse, Respirations
TURP	Transurethral Resection of Prostate
TX	Treatment
UA/C&S	Urinalysis/Culture and Sensitivity
UE	Upper Extremity
up ad lib	Up as Desired
UTI	Urinary Tract Infection
VNAA	Visiting Nurse Association of America
VO	Verbal Order
VS	Vital Signs
WIC	Women, Infants, & Children Program
WNL	Within Normal Limits

APPENDIX B

GLOSSARY OF TERMS

ACCREDITATION A rigorous process that examines various components of home care operations and clinical practice. The achievement of accreditation designates that the organization has gone through the accreditation process and meets predetermined standards as measured by onsite nurses and other survey team "visitors".

ACTIVITIES OF DAILY LIVING (ADL) Basic, usual self-care activities that must be done daily to care for our bodies and overall health. These activities include bathing, dressing, grooming, and toileting including clothing management and hygiene. ADL may also include simple meal preparation or doing laundry. These activities are important indicators because they demonstrate or show the patient's functional status or health care needs.

CAREGIVER Anyone who provides care or services to or for a patient.

CARE PLAN A plan of action for care that is developed, delivered, and evaluated by the nurse and other team members. This may also be called the plan of care and varies among organizations.

CASE MANAGEMENT A system for overseeing a patient's care usually across health care systems. For example, a nurse or therapist case manager may coordinate care and services from the hospital, to the nursing home, and in the patient's home.

CASE MANAGER One person who is responsible for the overall care of the patient and use of resources for that care. The case (or care) manager may be a nurse, a social worker, or a therapist.

CATHETER Any rounded or tubular medical device that is inserted into veins, cavities, or other body passages. The purpose of a catheter is to improve or replace function. Examples include a urinary foley catheter in the bladder from which urine drains into a collection bag, suction catheters, and intravenous catheters inserted into the vein which allow for the delivery of fluids.

CHRONIC A slow or persistent illness or health problem that must be cared for throughout life. Examples include diabetes, glaucoma, and some chronic lung conditions.

CLIENT The one who receives care. Also called the patient, customer, or consumer of health care services or products.

CLINICAL PATH (CP) A structured plan of care, oftentimes categorized by diagnosis or patient problem, that defines specific care interventions, team members, and other information across the timeline.

COLLABORATION The active process of working together and valuing another's input toward reaching patient goals.

CMS The Centers for Medicare and Medicaid Services. A part of the U.S. government that administers these health care insurance programs/benefits.

DEMENTIA Changes in brain function that cause memory loss, confusion, or the loss of ability to safely function independently.

DIAGNOSES The identification of problems or diseases. The word for one or a single diagnoses is diagnosis.

DIALYSIS The process of artificially cleansing the blood when the patient has renal or kidney failure. There are two kinds of dialysis, hemodialysis and peritoneal dialysis. For more information on how to care for a patient who receives dialysis, please see "Chronic Renal (Kidney) Failure".

DIETITIAN A member of the health care team who promotes optimal nutrition, based on the patient's individual needs. The dietitian may be called an R.D., a registered dietitian, or an L.D., a licensed dietitian. The dietitian may make home visits or teach the other team members about dietary related issues such as effective nutrition, meal preparation, and special diets.

DOCUMENTATION The writing of clinical notes that contains information needed for communication, legal, and other reasons. Documentation is completed in blue or black ink.

EDEMA Swelling in a particular part of the body. For example, the patient with swelling in the ankles or feet has edema and this should be reported to the nurse.

ENTERAL NUTRITION Provision of nourishment via a tube inserted into the nose and down to the stomach or through a surgical site through the stomach. A G-tube is an example of enteral nutrition.

G-TUBE A stomach or gastrostomy tube used to place nutrients into the stomach when the patient cannot safely swallow or eat.

GERIATRICS Services or care related or provided to older adults, related to the process of aging.

GOALS The endpoint of care or the desired results for care. For example, if the goal is to provide safe mobility, everything done should support that goal. The team members work to achieve the patient goals.

HOMEBOUND A term used in the Medicare home care program that means that the patient cannot leave the home without assistance and that leaving the home is a considerable and taxing effort and occurs infrequently and lasts for a short duration. Homebound means primarily confined to the home for medical reasons. "Homebound" is one of the admitting criteria for patients admitted to a Medicare certified home care program. For this reason, when patients are "no longer homebound", they are discharged from Medicare home health care.

HOME CARE/HOME HEALTH The provision of a range of health services, products, supplies and equipment to patients in their homes.

HOME HEALTH AGENCY An organization that provides care to patients in their homes. They may or may not be licensed, depending on the state and requirements. Medicare-certified agencies must have a survey or a special review to be certified to accept Medicare patients.

HOSPICE A special way of caring for patients with a terminal illness or a limited life expectancy. Hospice cares for the patient and their family and tries to make every remaining day the best that they can be. Hospice team members include specially trained hospice volunteers, bereavement counselors, certified nursing assistants (CNAs) or hospice aides, spiritual counselors, nurses, and other services. Hospice is a philosophy, not a place, but the bulk of hospice care is provided at home.

LARYNGECTOMY Surgical removal of the voicebox resulting in the loss of normal speech ability.

MEDICAID A health program that is administered at the state level for patients who qualify. The qualification is financial. Medicaid coverage varies by state. Sometimes even the name is different. For example, in California it is called Medical.

MEDICARE A federal program for people over age 65, the disabled, or those who have end stage renal disease (ESRD). Medicare is complex and has different parts that cover different services such as inpatient hospitalization (after the Medicare beneficiary pays a deductible), home care, hospice, and other services. Medicare is a medical insurance program, and like all insurance programs there are exclusions, eligibility, and coverage rules. The Centers for Medicare and Medicaid Services (CMS) administer the programs. The CMS is a part of the Health and Human Services (HHS) administration of the government.

OCCUPATIONAL SAFETY AND HEALTH ADMINIS-TRATION (OSHA) The part of the U.S. Government that regulates employee or worker safety. OSHA requires various standards be maintained related to health care.

OCCUPATIONAL THERAPY Occupational therapy (OT) is the use of therapeutic activity and exercise to help individuals with limitations to function as safely and independently as possible. The OT teaches use of compensating techniques and assistive devices to improve their ability to perform self-care and other ADL such as bathing, meal preparation, etc.

OUTCOMES Outcomes are quantifiable or measurable goals of care. An example is the patient, by a certain date, can name all of their medications, and the time to take them. Outcomes are usually measured across points in time.

PARAPLEGIA Paralysis or loss of motor ability of the lower extremities or legs.

PARENTERAL NUTRITION The provision of nourishment via an intravenous (IV) route.

PAYOR The payor or insurance company financially responsible for the services or care provided to patients. Examples include Medicare or other insurance companies.

PEDIATRIC OR PEDIATRICS Services or care related to children. Pediatrics is a specialty that involves the development, care, and problems or disease of children and childhood. This includes newborns, infants, toddlers, and all ages of children through adolescence.

PERFORMANCE IMPROVEMENT An ongoing process that seeks to continuously improve patient care, delivery of services, staff education, and other important parts of operations or other parts of an organization. Accreditation standards demand continuous quality improvement. Home care or hospice aides may be involved in various parts of CQI or be asked to serve on certain committees.

PERSONAL EMERGENCY RESPONSE SYSTEM (PERS) A technology that links the frail or homebound to community resources in the case of a fall or other emergency. PERS usually have a personal help button which when activated, calls for help. To be effective, the PERS personal help button must be worn, carried, or within reach at all times.

PHYSICAL THERAPY (PT) A specialty of the rehabilitation services that focuses on mobility and function of patients due to illness or injury. Physical therapists or PTs work with stroke patients, patients with impairments to legs or back, and others who need home exercises or other programs to restore safe mobility and function.

QUADRIPLEGIA Paralysis or loss of motor ability of all upper and lower extremities, both arms and legs. This is also called tetraplegia.

REHABILITATION The term used to describe the care and efforts of team members to restore function and mobility after illness or injury. Members of the rehabilitation team include the physical therapist, occupational therapist, and speech-language pathologist. The aide may have assignments related to the patient's rehabilitation that the therapist or nurse may assign, based on the patient's individualized rehabilitation program and other needs.

SOCIAL WORK SERVICES (SWS) Social work services, also called medical social services (MSS), are valuable services to patients and their families for a number of reasons. The social worker or medical social worker (MSW)may be involved when there are problems that prevent the plan of care from being implemented. For example, if the patient has diabetes and cannot afford food or insulin, or if there are family or other problems that are causing the patient not to improve or be in unsafe conditions.

SPEECH-LANGUAGE PATHOLOGY (SLP) The speech-language pathologist or speech therapist is involved primarily with patients who have swallowing or communication problems after surgery or due to other problems such as a stroke.

SUPERVISORY VISIT Supervisory Visits are requirements of Medicare. The nurse may visit sometimes when the HHA is providing care in the home and other times when the aide is not at the home. Supervision is a standard practice in home and hospice care and assists in assuring quality of care for patients.

RESPIRATORY THERAPY The respiratory therapist is a specialist usually involved with patients who need oxygen or have other respiratory problems or illnesses.

TRACHEOSTOMY Surgical creation of an opening in the skin to the trachea, the breathing tube.

VENIPUNCTURE A puncture into the vein to draw blood. The nurse or lab technician obtains blood through venipuncture for laboratory analysis.

APPENDIX C

EXAMPLE OF A HOME HEALTH AIDE PERFORMANCE EVALUATION

This is an example of the kinds of information that contributes to the home health aide's performance evaluation or appraisal of performance. As an employee, the aide's performance will be evaluated.

1) Is the home health aide following infection control standards as defined by the organization's policies and procedures?

2) Is the home health aide using safe body mechanics, as defined by the organization's policies and procedures? (Examples could include use of lumbar support belt, correct lifting, etc.)

3) Is the home health aide adhering to the organization's policy related to dress code and appearance?

4) Is the home health aide at the client's home as scheduled?

5) Does the home health aide consistently and correctly contact the supervisor for scheduling delays or problems?

6) Does the home health aide consistently promote home safety according to the organization's policies and procedures?

7) Does the home health aide demonstrate effective communication and other skills with the patient and their family?

8) Does the home health aide submit complete, legible, accurate documentation in a timely manner?

9) Other questions, as defined by the organization.

Recommendations for Improvement:

____

____

____

____

____

____

Corrective Action/Follow-up:

____

____

____

____

____

____

APPENDIX D

EDUCATIONAL RESOURCES

ASSOCIATIONS

Most of the states have a home care and a hospice state association. In some states, such as New Mexico, there is one state association for both home care and hospice organizations. These state associations are very important for knowing state regulations and requirements as well as for networking and ongoing education.

The National Association for Home Care and Hospice (NAHC) can be reached by calling (202) 547-7424 or by visiting **http://www.nahc.org**.

The National Hospice and Palliative Care Organization (NHPCO). The NHPCO offers a Certified Nursing Assistant (CAN) Section and Leader that represents the CNAs in hospice. For information about individual Council of Hospice Professionals membership, call (703) 243-5900. The NHPCO's website is located at **http://www.nhpco.org**.

The National Private Duty Association. Can be reached by calling (317) 663-3637, or email at **info@privatedutyhomecare.org** or visit their website at **www.privatedutyhomecare.org**

The Visiting Nurse Associations of America (VNAA) can be reached by calling (617) 737-3200. The VNAA website is **http://www.vnaa.org**.

The Hospice and Palliative Nurses Association (HPNA) offers membership and certification for home health aides and certified nursing assistants. For information, call (412) 787-9301 or visit their website at **http://www.hpna.org**.

BOOKS

Birchenall, J., Straight, E. (2003). *Mosby's Textbook for the Home Care Aide.* St. Louis, MO: Mosby.

Falvo, Donna R. (2004). *Effective Patient Education: A Guide to Increased Compliance, Third Edition.* Sudbury, MA: Jones and Bartlett Publishers.

Fuzy, J. (2000). *The Home Health Aide Handbook.* Hartman Publishing.

Mace, N.L., and Rabins, P. (1991). *The 36 Hour Day: A Family Guide to Caring for Persons with Alzheimer Disease and Related Dementing Illness and Memory Loss Later in Life.* Baltimore, MD: Johns Hopkins University Press. To order call (800) 537-5487.

Marrelli, T.M. *Handbook of Home Health Standards and Documentation Guidelines for Reimbursement.* St. Louis, MO: Mosby. To order call (800) 993-6397.

Marrelli, T.M. (2008). *Home Health Aide: Guidelines for Care - - Instructor Manual, Second Edition.* To order, call (800) 993-6397or visit http://www.marrelli.com.

Marrelli, T.M. (2005). *Hospice and Palliative Care Handbook: Quality, Compliance, and Reimbursement, Second Edition.* Mosby. To order, call (800) 993-6397 or visit http://www.marrelli.com.

Redman, Barbara Klug. (2001). *The Practice of Patient Education, Ninth Edition.* St. Louis, MO: Mosby.

Williams, M. (2001). *Q + A Review for Home Care Aide.* Prentice Hall.

NEWSLETTERS

Home Health Aide Digest is a subscription newsletter published six times a year dedicated to nurturing the occupational and personal growth of home health aides. To review a copy call (800) 340-3356 or visit their website at **http://www.hhadigest.com.**

SERVICES

Marrelli and Associates, Inc. provides consultative services to home care and hospice programs. Individualized seminars are available for home care or hospice organizations, which include training on documentation requirements, clinical paths, and many others. For information call (800) 993-6397 or visit http://www.marrelli.com.

SUPPLIES/FORMS

Briggs Corporation provides products for both home care and hospice through their website at **http://www.briggscorp.com** or call them at (877) 307-1744.

Hopkins Medical Products website catalog can be viewed online or can be reached by calling (800) 835-1995 or, to view the catalog and order online, visit their website at **http://www.hopkinsmedicalproducts.com.**

Med-Pass offers many documentation and reference products for home health care and hospice care. They can be reached at (800) 438-8884 or by visiting their website at **http://www.med-pass.com.**

APPENDIX E

Home Health Aide Coverage of Services (CMS Publication 11, The Home Health Agency Manual)

206.2 <u>Home Health Aide Services.</u>— For home health aide services to be covered, the patient must meet the qualifying criteria as specified in §204, the services provided by the home health aide must be part-time or intermittent as discussed in §206.7; the services must meet the definition of home health aide services of this section; and the services must be reasonable and necessary to the treatment of the patient's illness or injury.

The reason for the visits by the home health aide must be to provide hands-on personal care to the patient or services that are needed to maintain the patient's health or to facilitate treatment of the patient's illness or injury.

The physician's order should indicate the frequency of the home health aide services required by the patient. These services may include but are not limited to:

a. <u>Personal Care.</u>—Personal care means:

o Bathing, dressing, grooming, caring for hair, nail and oral hygiene that are needed to facilitate treatment or prevent deterioration of the patient's health, changing the bed linens of an incontinent patient, shaving, deodorant application, skin care with lotions and/or powder, foot care, and ear care.

o Feeding, assistance with elimination (including enemas unless the skills of a licensed nurse are required due to the patient's condition), routine catheter care and routine colostomy care, assistance with ambulation, changing position in bed, assistance with transfers.

EXAMPLE 1: A physician has ordered home health aide visits to assist the patient in personal care because the patient is recovering from a stroke and continues to have significant right side weakness that causes him to be unable to bathe, dress or perform hair and oral care. The plan of care established by the HHA nurse sets forth the specific tasks with which the patient needs assistance. Home health aide visits at an appropriate frequency would be reasonable and necessary to assist in these tasks.

EXAMPLE 2: A physician ordered four home health aide visits per week for personal care for a multiple sclerosis patient who is unable to perform these functions because of increasing debilitation. The home health aide gave the patient a bath twice per week and washed hair on the other two visits each week. Only two visits are reasonable and necessary since the services could have been provided in the course of two visits.

EXAMPLE 3: A physician ordered seven home health aide visits per week for personal care for a bed-bound, incontinent patient. All visits are reasonable and necessary because the patient has extensive personal care needs.

EXAMPLE 4: A patient with a well-established colostomy forgets to change the bag regularly and has difficulty changing the bag. Home health aide services at an appropriate frequency to change the bag would be considered reasonable and necessary to the treatment of the illness or injury.

b. Simple dressing changes that do not require the skills of a licensed nurse.

EXAMPLE: A patient who is confined to the bed has developed a small-reddened area on the buttocks. The physician has ordered home health aide visits for more frequent repositioning, bathing and the application of a topical ointment and a gauze 4x4. Home health aide visits at an appropriate frequency would be reasonable and necessary.

c. Assistance with medications that are ordinarily self-administered and do not require the skills of a licensed nurse to be provided safely and effectively.

NOTE: Prefilling of insulin syringes is ordinarily performed by the diabetic as part of the self-administration of the insulin and, unlike the injection of the insulin, does not require the skill of a licensed nurse to be performed properly. Therefore, if the prefilling of insulin syringes is performed by HHA staff, it is considered to be a home health aide service. However, where State law precludes the provision of this service by other than a licensed nurse or physician, Medicare will make payment for this service, when covered, as though it were a skilled nursing service. Where the patient needs only prefilling of insulin syringes and does not need skilled nursing care on an intermittent basis, physical therapy or speech-language pathology services or have a continuing need for occupational therapy, then Medicare cannot cover any home health services to the patient (even if State law requires that the insulin syringes be filled by a licensed nurse).

Home health aide services are those services ordered in the plan of care that the aide is permitted to perform under State law. Medicare coverage of the administration of insulin by a home health aide will depend on whether or not the agency is in compliance with all Federal and State laws and regulations related to this task. However, when the task of insulin administration has been delegated to the home health aide, the task must be considered and billed as a Medicare home health aide service. By a State allowing the delegation of insulin administration to home health aides, the State has extended the role of aides, not equated aide services with the services of a registered nurse.

d. Assistance with activities that are directly supportive of skilled therapy services but do not require the skills of a therapist to be safely and effectively performed such as routine maintenance exercises, and repetitive practice of functional communication skills to support speech-language pathology services.

e. Routine care of prosthetic and orthotic devices. When a home health aide visits a patient to provide a health related service as discussed above, the home health aide may also perform some incidental services that do not meet the definition of a home health aide service (e.g., light cleaning, preparation of a meal, taking out the trash, shopping). However, the purpose of a home health aide visit may not be to provide these incidental services since they are not health related services, but rather are necessary household tasks that must be performed by anyone to maintain a home.

EXAMPLE 1: A home health aide visits a recovering stroke patient whose right side weakness and poor endurance cause her to be able to leave the bed and chair only with extreme difficulty. The physician has ordered physical therapy and speech-language pathology services for the patient and has ordered home health aide services three or four times per week for personal care, assistance with ambulation as mobility increases, and assistance with repetitive speech exercises as her impaired speech improves. The home health aide also provides incidental household services such as preparation of meals, light cleaning and taking out the trash. The patient lives with an elderly frail sister who is disabled and cannot perform either the personal care or the incidental tasks. The home health aide visits at a frequency appropriate to the performance of the health related services would be covered, notwithstanding the incidental provision of noncovered services (i.e., the household services) in the course of the visits.

EXAMPLE 2: A physician orders home health aide visits three times per week. The only services provided are light housecleaning, meal preparation and trash removal. The home health aide visits cannot be covered, notwithstanding their importance to the patient, because the services provided do not meet Medicare's definition of "home health aide services."

206.3 <u>Medical Social Services.</u>—Medical social services that are provided by a qualified medical social worker or a social work assistant under the supervision of a qualified medical social worker may be covered as home health services where the patient meets the qualifying criteria specified in §204, and:

- The services of these professionals are necessary to resolve social or emotional problems that are or are expected to be an impediment to the effective treatment of the patient's medical condition or his or her rate of recovery; and:
- The plan of care indicates how the services that are required necessitate the skills of a qualified social worker or a social work assistant under the supervision of a qualified medical social worker to be performed safely and effectively.
- Where both of these requirements for coverage are met, services of these professionals that may be covered include, but are not limited to:
- Assessment of the social and emotional factors related to the patient's illness, need for care, response to treatment and adjustment to care;
- Assessment of the relationship of the patient's

medical and nursing requirements to the patient's home situation, financial resources and availability of community resources;

- Appropriate action to obtain available community resources to assist in resolving the patient's problem. (Note: Medicare does not cover the services of a medical social worker to complete or assist in the completion of an application for Medicaid because Federal regulations require the State to provide assistance in completing the application to anyone who chooses to apply for Medicaid.);
- Counseling services which are required by the patient

484.36

(d) Standard: Supervision

1) If the patient receives skilled nursing care, the registered nurse must perform the supervisory visit required by paragraph (d) of this section. If the patient is not receiving skilled nursing care, but is receiving another skilled service (that is, physical therapy, occupational therapy, or speech-language pathology services), supervision may be provided by the appropriate therapist.

2) The registered nurse (or other professional described in paragraph (d)(1) of this section must make an on-site visit to the patient's home no less frequently than every two weeks.

If home health aide services are provided to a patient who is not receiving skilled nursing care, physical, or occupational therapy or speech-language pathology services, the registered nurse must make a supervisory visit to the patient's home no less frequently than every 60 days. In these cases, to ensure that the aide is properly caring for the patient, each supervisory visit must occur while the home health aide is providing patient care.

APPENDIX F

Home Health Aide and Homemaker Coverage of Services (CMS Publication 21, The Medicare Hospice Manual)

230.1 (Cont.) General inpatient care under the hospice benefit is not equivalent to a hospital level of care under the Medicare hospital benefit. For example, a brief period of general inpatient care may be needed in some cases when a patient elects the hospice benefit at the end of a covered hospital stay. If a patient in this circumstance continues to need pain control or symptom management which cannot be feasibly provided in other settings while he or she prepares to receive hospice home care, general inpatient care is appropriate.

Other examples of appropriate general inpatient care include a patient in need of medication adjustment, observation, or other stabilizing treatment, such as psycho-social monitoring, or a patient whose family is unwilling to permit needed care to be furnished in the home.

Inpatient respite care may be furnished to provide respite for the individual's family or other persons caring for the individual at home.

Note that hospice inpatient care in an SNF or NF serves to prolong current benefit periods for general Medicare hospital and SNF benefits. This could potentially affect patients who revoke the hospice benefit.

F. <u>Medical Appliances and Supplies, Including Drugs and Biologicals.</u>— Only drugs as defined in §1861(t) of the Act and which are used primarily for the relief of pain and symptom control related to the individual's terminal illness are covered. Appliances include covered durable medical equipment as described in 42 CFR 410.38 as well as other self-help and personal comfort items related to the palliation or management of the patient's terminal illness. Equipment is provided by the hospice for use in the patient's home while he or she is under hospice care. Medical supplies include those that are part of the written plan of care.

G. <u>Home Health Aide and Homemaker Services.</u>—Home health aide services may only be provided by individuals who have successfully completed a home health aide training and competency evaluation program or competency evaluation program as required in 42 CFR 484.36. Home health aides may provide personal care services. Aides may also perform household services to maintain a safe and sanitary environment in areas of the home used by the patient, such as changing the bed or light cleaning and laundering essential to the comfort and cleanliness of the patient. Aide services must be provided under the general supervision of a registered nurse. Homemaker services may include assistance in personal care, maintenance of a safe and healthy environment and services to enable the individual to carry out the plan of care.

H. <u>Physical Therapy, Occupational Therapy and Speech-Language Pathology Services.</u>—Therapy and speech-language pathology services may be provided for purposes of symptom control or to enable the individual to maintain activities of daily living and basic functional skills.

INDEX

C

Calling in sick, 18
Cancer, 117-119
  breast, 114-116
Canes, quad
  after hip fractures, 107, 108
  assistance with, 7
Capability, of HHAs, 19-20
Car insurance, requirements for, 83
Car safety, 66
Cardiac care patients, 120-122
  see also Heart failure (HF)
Cardiac medications, 120, 121
Cardiopulmonary resuscitation (CPR)
  certification, requirements for, 83
Cardiovascular disease;
  see Cardiac care patients
Care, refusal of, in patients' bill of
  rights, 20
Care coordination, 43
Caregivers; see also Families changes
  in, reporting of, 27 support of,
  Alzheimer's disease and, 98
Caregiving skills, clinical, 5
Caring behaviors, 8-9, 21
Case coordination;
  see Care coordination
Catheters
  care of, 7, 134
  urinary, see Urinary catheters
Cerebral vascular accidents
  (CVAs), 123-126
  communication problems after, 20
Certificates, for continuing
  education, 83
Certification, organizational, 50
Certified nursing assistants
  (CNAs), 156
Certified occupational therapy
  assistants (COTA), in home care, 38
Changes
  in patients condition, reporting,
  25-27, 39, 40, 46
  in scheduling, 61
CHAP, 53
Chemotherapy, as treatment for
  cancer, 118
Chest pains; see Cardiac care patients
Children, care of, 127-128
Chocolate, diabetes and, 32

Chronic lung disease, see Lung
  diseases, chronic
Chronic obstructive pulmonary
  disease (COPD), 129-132
Chronic renal failure, 133-135
Circulation, of diabetic patients,
  142-145
Cleaning, 8
  equipment, 75, 130
  of patient care area, 75-76
Cleaning liquids, for infection
  control, 72
Clinical caregiving skills, 4
Clinical documentation; see
  Documentation
CNAs, 156
Colds, infection control and, 72-73
Colostomy care, 7, see also Cancer
Comfort measures, 8
Commodes, 7
Communication, 5, see also Teams
  of changes in patient status, 25-27
  with depressed patients, 140
  explaining procedures, 9
  language differences, 20
  negative, 43-44
  nonverbal; see Nonverbal
    communication
  with organization, 12
  with patients/families, on teams,
  46-47
  of scheduling changes, 61
  with supervisors, 9,11
Communication difficulties,
  of patients, 20-21
Community Health Accreditation
  Program (CHAP), 53
Compatibility, with patients, 17-18
Competency evaluations, 5
Complaints, reporting of, 26
Conferences, of teams, 44-46
Confidence, of HHAs, 24
Confidentiality, 3, 6, 9, 20, 31, 47
  in patients' bill of rights, 30
Confusion states; see Alzheimer's
  disease
Congestive heart failure (HF),
  see also Cardiac care patients
Constipation, 136-138
  in hospice care, 158,159
Continuing education, 5
  certificates for, 83

NOTES AND PHONE NUMBERS

NOTES AND PHONE NUMBERS

NOTES AND PHONE NUMBERS

QUICK ORDER FORM

Telephone Orders: (941) 697-290(
(800) 993-NEWS (6397

Fax Orders: (941) 697-2901
Copy and send this form

Mail Orders: Marrelli and Associates, Inc.,
P.O. Box 629, Boca Grande, FL
33921-0629

E-mail Orders: *news@marrelli.com, www.marrelli.com*

Please send the following book:

Home Health Aide: Guidelines for Care A Handbook for Caregiving at Home (2007)

$29.95 ea. x __________ = __________
($26.95 + $3 s/h)   Books   Total

Home Health Aide: Guidelines for Care Instructor Manual (2007)

$179.95 ea. x __________ = __________
($169.95 + $10 s/h)   Manuals   Total

Please send FREE information on:

□ *Other books*   □ *Speaking/ Seminars*   □ *Consulting*   □ *Home Healthcare Nurse*
(Journal Issue)

Name:____

Organization:_________________________________

Address:______________________________________

□ Office Address   □ Home Address

City: ____________________________ **State:**_________

Zip:__________

Telephone:___________________________________

Fax:____

E-mail:______________________________________

Sales Tax: Please add 7% sales tax on orders shipped to Florida addresses.

Payment: □ Check   □ Credit Card   □ Amex

            □ Visa   □ MasterCard

Card Number: __________________________ **Exp:** _____/____

Name on card: __________________________________

Cardholder's Signature: ___________________________

Visit Marrelli and Associates, Inc. on the World Wide Web at www.marrelli.com